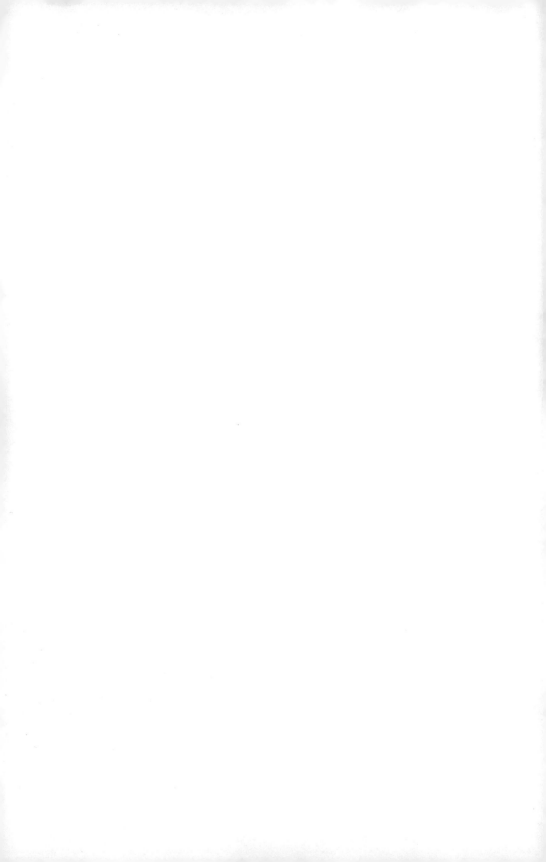

FERTILE GROUND

FERTILE GROUND

WOMEN, EARTH, AND THE LIMITS OF CONTROL

IRENE DIAMOND

BEACON PRESS
BOSTON

Beacon Press
25 Beacon Street
Boston, Massachusetts 02108-2892

Beacon Press books
are published under the auspices of
the Unitarian Universalist Association of Congregations.

99 98 97 96 95 94   8 7 6 5 4 3 2 1

Text design by Ruth Kolbert

Library of Congress Cataloging-in-Publication Data

Diamond, Irene, 1947–
Fertile ground : women, earth, and the limits of control /
Irene Diamond.
p.   cm.
Includes bibliographical references and index.
ISBN 0-8070-6772-5
1. Ecofeminism.   2. Birth control—Social aspects.   3. Fertility,
Human—Social aspects.   I. Title.
HQ1233.D5   1994
304.6′32—dc20   93-39064
CIP

*This book is dedicated to the memory
of my grandmother, Hayah Sarah Orinofsky,
my mother, Esther Frieda Grossman,
and to the visions of my partner in life and work, Jeff Land,
and our daughter, Maya.*

CONTENTS

CONTENTS

FOREWORD

Even social movements that are effective at bringing about change encounter limitations imposed by their own blind spots, the assumptions and premises that are not noticed because they themselves form the frame through which adherents look. Thus classical Marxism, embedded in the mechanistic model of nineteenth century science, could ignore issues of ecology and environmental damage, as some groups within the environmental movement today ignore issues of gender. What we do see—the problems we can identify, the destruction we can name, the hope we can articulate—moves us forward, until we run up against the invisible bars of what we *don't* see and begin to hear the challenges of those who have been voiceless.

The primary insight of ecofeminism is that all issues of oppression are interconnected, that to understand how to heal and liberate our world, we must look at the relationships between the various systems by which power is constructed. In an ecofeminist vision, there is no such thing as a struggle for women's rights separate from a struggle to repair the living systems of the earth that sustain life, or a struggle for gender equality that can be divided from a struggle for equality along lines of race, culture, economics, ancestry, religion, sexual orientation, or physical ability.

In *Fertile Ground,* Irene Diamond has written a passionate and provocative book that challenges the feminist movement to step beyond its preconceptions. She identifies one of our primary blind spots—the use of the language of control. In a world of media sound bites and twenty-second interviews, political movements are necessarily forced to simplify, to reduce complex issues to slogans and catchy phrases. But Diamond identifies the toll this takes on the feminist imagination.

One insight shared by deconstructionists and Witches is that language shapes reality. Or rather, we might say that language determines the latitude of our responses to the challenges reality presents. When feminists adopt the language of control, we have already limited the range of our vision and locked ourselves into a worldview that may not serve our truest ends.

What we need and want, as women, is freedom from external control, not to be forced to put our sexuality or our powers of reproduction at the service of others' ends. But when we speak of "the right to control our bodies," or "the right to control our fertility," we have unconsciously accepted the oppressive core assumption of modern culture—that the body can be and should be controlled, that the mysteries of the kindling of life and the awakening of desire and the formation of one being out of another, the great processes of birth and growth and decay and death, are ultimately knowable and controllable.

That unacknowledged acceptance of control as a value insidiously shapes our thinking, about women's bodies, about the earth and our relationship to all the living systems that sustain life, about what ends are desirable and what means are acceptable. It narrows the discourse about issues that are complex and emotional, such as abortion and the new technologies of fertility, locks us into battling on narrow ramparts, and abandons the terrain of the sacred to the right-wing fundamentalists.

Diamond documents the way that this same language imposes structures of control on the most vulnerable women, those of the third world and of indigenous cultures, whose own organic worldview is discounted as the land itself is sacrificed to the 'control' of technologies that ultimately destroy it. And she leaves us with hope, embodied in the self-organized movements of women around the world, informed and empowered by their direct connection with and dependence on the basic elements of life—seeds and soil, water, fire, and air.

Fertile Ground is sure to be controversial, for it breaks through the accepted boundaries of thought and dares to suggest that both politics and academia need to grapple with the questions of deep value we call questions of the sacred. To many feminists, this is heresy. To the deep ecologists, who have raised this same issue in the environmental movement, her arguments may sound too human—centered, too culturally focused. But the brilliance of her argument is that she grapples with the mysteries without losing sight of the very human structures of language and power which need to change in order to heal our relationships with each other and with the natural world. We desperately need this synthesis. We need to imagine a politics that can counter structures of control without imposing new, more subtle forms of domination. We need to become more comfortable with the language of mystery than with the language of control, not to abandon the rational but to temper it with the ability to stand in reverent wonder at the cycles of birth, growth, death, and rebirth as they play themselves out in our bodies and the world around us. Only then can our political movements, our technologies, and our knowledge move us beyond the constraints of our thinking into the free air where we can learn to heal the damage, share the wealth, and survive.

STARHAWK

PREFACE

*Western culture is in the middle of a fundamental transformation;
a "shape of life" is growing old. The demise of the old is being
hastened by the end of colonialism, the uprising of women, the
revolt of other cultures against white Western hegemony, shifts in
the balance of economic and political power within the world
economy, and a growing awareness of the costs as well as the
benefits of scientific and technological "progress." . . . recent
events in Western history have posed fundamental challenges to
the self-certainty of reason and its "science." The anti-Enlighten-
ment cranks now seem more like prophets. It is no longer self-
evident that there is any necessary connection between reason,
knowledge, science, freedom, and human happiness.*

JANE FLAX,
Thinking Fragments

*The culture of the technological age has successfully gripped
men's minds by reprocessing and repackaging our conception of
history into a neat dichotomy in which technology is the future
and all previous civilisations fade into the irrelevant past.*

APARNA VISWANTHAN,
The Times of India

*Diversity, generally understood and embraced, is not casual
liberal tolerance of anything and everything not yourself. It is
not polite accommodation. Instead, diversity is, in action, the
sometimes painful awareness that other people, other races,
other voices, other habits of mind, have as much integrity of
being, as much claim on the world as you do. . . . And I urge you,
amid all the differences present to the eye and mind, to reach out
to create the bond that . . . will protect us all. We are meant to be
here together.*

WILLIAM M. CHASE,
The Language of Action

THIS HAS BEEN A HARD BOOK TO WRITE. IT QUESTIONS a tenet of the contemporary feminist movement so pervasive that to scrutinize it is to seemingly question feminism itself: the assumption that a woman's freedom lies in the right to gain control over her body and sexuality. Yet I have come to believe that this stance contains certain contradictions and dangers, problems which become evident from what I call an ecofeminist perspective. Ecofeminists, through their insistence on our connection to all forms of life, their refusal to accept the dominant culture's limited approach to knowing, and their practice in which the struggle to empower women and the struggle to save the planet are joined, celebrate rather than fear our dependence on a living fertile earth.

I did not arrive at this understanding all at once. Much of this book charts the fits and starts whereby I came to recognize the inadequacies of the principles, practices, and modes of knowing which once made a great deal of sense to me. For over a decade my interrogation of the right to control our bodies has often made me uncomfortable with the stances of feminist leaders, medical experts, and some of my dearest friends take. In claiming that fertility, human and vegetative, is threatened by the underlying instrumentalism the Western will to mastery intends, I am arguing that feminists and others might well be served by a new ethic that respects spontaneity, reciprocity, and yes, even mystery.

This book does not provide a simple or obvious answer for dealing with the technologies of the contemporary world. Throughout, I invoke a politics of resistance, but I am mindful of how difficult that can often be in practice. The enticements of modern life confound even the most critical assessments of their baleful effects. As I type this on my computer I realize that in some basic ways this book would not have been possible without some of the most pervasive of those tools it seemingly indicts. I have had to agonize over my own practices more times than I wished.

This book would have been difficult enough had I simply chosen to reinterpret feminism from an ecological perspective. However, my commitment to the deeply humane and affirmative visions of feminism has led me to engage the morally, historically, and scientifically problematic approach to the so-called population problem that permeates the modern environmental movement as well. The questioning that informs this book is influenced by the writings of the late Michel Foucault, from whom I take seriously the proposition that language constructs our world. As a consequence I do not readily accept such standard categories of analysis as "carrying capacity," "resources," and "population," which many ecologists tend to assume simply inhere in the world. The environmental movement's fixation on the image of teeming masses devouring limited resources has inspired many to actions I often applaud, but the image is reductive and reinforces a grievously limited understanding of the peoples and cultures that preceded us as well as of how we might repair the devastation that has been wrought by scientific certainty and the modern state system. The apocalyptic thinking that infuses the modern environmental movement is the alarmed response to this pervasive image of a shrinking planet overrun and consumed by human bodies. I worry both about the consequences that flow from the image and the apocalyptic thinking. Thus, this book questions certain of the central beliefs of those movements with which I am most engaged.

Though I am joyous that both women and men are beginning to rediscover the intricate webs of connection between the well-being of our bodies and the well-being of our precious earth, connections that indigenous cultures through time have made, I am also a bit cautious. My caution stems from my sense that while on one level the wisdom we need is but the simple ethical one encapsulated in Gandhi's famous words that "the world provides enough for everyone's needs, but not enough for everyone's greed," our failure to heed this wisdom results in part from the influence of our culture's ideology of control. Relearning and reimagining is absolutely vital, and it is my fervent wish that what I have learned in the course of writing this book can make a small contribution to these endeavors.

In the course of writing this book I have encountered many people who honor the simple ecological wisdom "we are made from this earth" as they struggle for the highest ideals of democracy and social justice. They have inspired this book. And however challenging the writing of *Fertile Ground* has been, it has been made easier by the friends and compatriots who stood by me through the duration, encouraging me to continue what at times seemed a never-ending project.

I am particularly endebted to Lee Quinby for conversations over the years. Our work together on Foucault was crucial to the evolution of this book. Gloria Orenstein, Charlotte Talberth, and Gail Omvedt were essential guides in my different journeys toward ecological awareness. Lois Banner, Sarah Douglas, Phil Green, Miriam Johnson, Cheris Kramarae, Jane Mansbridge, Barbara Pope, Cheyney Ryan, and John Stuhr took the time to read portions of the manuscript in its different incarnations. I must also thank Dick Kraus and Brian Tokar who guided me to crucial materials and the anonymous reviewers who offered insightful critiques. Danny Moses, Charlene Spretnak, and Diana Sheridan nourished my spirit. Mark Jeffries and Joan-Marie Michaelson helped with various aspects of the research. Marna Hauck's intelligence and energy got me through some difficult times. My sons, Ross and Adam, assisted in innumerable ways from the beginning until the end.

A special thanks to the staff at Beacon. They were much wiser than I about the title. The late Deborah Johnson incubated the manuscript during its initial stages. The book was guided to completion under the astute criticism of Lauren Bryant. No one could ask for a more attentive, intelligent, and sensitive editor. Without the unflagging support and wise counsel of my husband, Jeffrey, this book could not have been written.

The initial stage of this project was supported by a fellowship from the American Association of University Women. Other support was provided by the Oregon Committee for the Humanities and both the Humanities Center and the Center for Research for Women in Society at the University of Oregon. The Fulbright Association of India made it possible for me to do research there during 1991–92.

FEMINISM,
FERTILITY,
AND THE
LIVING EARTH

Clever animals though we remain, our culture remains, our civilization remains, very much a creation of the soil we live on. No more than we ever could, can we afford exhaustive use—which is abuse—of fertility.

EDWARD HYAMS,
Soil and Civilization

We must create new images to convey our visions, and to do so we must be patient (though not passive), for images will not be called into being by sheer acts of will alone. Rather we learn what artists know well: that authentic images arise from our unconscious as gifts; that out of our living, from our whole, engaged selves, with the support of our communities, the images that serve us will emerge. We must trust the journey. There are no shortcuts.

MARCIA FALK,
"Notes on Composing New Blessings"

*now
while greed, lust, terror, shame
rule our lives
forgotten goddesses return
to heal, to care
to create
to celebrate
to reclaim the earth
for all of us*

VIMOCHANA,
Forum for Women's Rights

THE HOPE THAT THE EARTH MIGHT BE RECLAIMED for all grows from the basic wisdom that to reclaim the earth we need to recreate ourselves. We must reimagine who we are as persons and create an appropriate politics. This difficult task becomes ever more urgent as doomsayers insist there will soon be no earth to reclaim if human "population" is not drastically curbed and controlled. At the same time, the cacophony of voices from cultures colonized by white European adventurers emphasize their unique histories. Recognition of a common terrain seems ever more tenuous.

I come to these complicated issues as a feminist of North America whose ecological sensibilities are recently formed. I have few tales of feeling a connection with the living earth. Growing up in New Jersey in the 1950s, I was two generations and thousands of miles removed from my Russian heritage. New York City was the center of my universe. I was mostly impressed with the cleverness of human artifice and indeed had no sense of myself as having any particular kinship to the natural world, as being a creature "of the soil." I had no favorite childhood tree or stream and was most comfortable viewing animals behind the safety of the guard rails in the Bronx Zoo. Mountains were the Catskills, where one played games around a concrete swimming pool.

Knowledge was something obtained from books or from questioning those who had read more books than I had.

In 1968, when I was pregnant for the first time, I readily agreed to be put to sleep for the birth of my child. I "chose" this mode of delivery not because I was especially cowed by medical authority or because there was anything especially unusual about the pregnancy, but simply because I had no particular thoughts or feelings on the matter. My response to the obstetrician's inquiry as to what type of delivery I wanted was to ask what he preferred. My concerns was to make sure he had no problems with my plan to go straight on to graduate school. (As an only child with little knowledge of babies, I was not daunted, indeed took little note, that the catalogue had said admissions preference would be given to qualified young men). I prepared for childbirth and graduate school by reading books on African politics.

By the time of my second pregnancy in 1970 my identity was fully tied up in feminism. There was no question that this time around I would not be comatose during childbirth and would prepare for the more "natural" birthing feminists were struggling to reclaim. Friends wondered why I didn't extend this logic to include breastfeeding and I responded with my worries about maintaining equality in parenting. Though I eventually decided that equality did not preclude breastfeeding, I also insisted on keeping myself to a dissertation regimen that made no accommodation to the physical demands of nursing. A commitment to public activities and geographic mobility with respect to career options were my ideals. Caught up in the sexual and contraceptive revolutions I switched from the pill to the I.U.D., with the thought that a diaphragm was not a choice because it would intrude on sexual pleasure, not permitting me to be as spontaneous and carefree as men.

By the second half of the seventies, I'd grown increasingly conscious of the problem of male behavior as the standard truth. I began to ponder the dynamics of the sexual revolution I and my contemporaries had experienced. Yes, there were the powerful discoveries of new pleasures, but why did it feel that men's notions of commitment and fidelity had somehow won the day? Had women been full and equal participants in setting the terms of the new arrangements? Had liberation mostly created new pressures and new opportunities for women to conform to men's fantasies and wants?

In the midst of this questioning of sexual practices I found myself organizing a demonstration in 1976 against a photographer from *Playboy* magazine who had come to Purdue University to photograph "girls of the Big 10." Soon after I began to think about the subject of pornography and the media's exploitation of women's bodies. Angered by the blatant misogyny of snuff movies and billboards and record jackets depicting bound women being tortured, I began to challenge the notion that pornography was harmless and unrelated to crimes against women. In 1978, at the Feminist Perspectives on Pornography conference, in San Francisco I walked with other women in the first Take Back the Night March in the United States to express our outrage about sexual violence.[1] Three years later I traveled to Denmark with my two young sons to try to figure out what really happened when the Danes legalized pornography. Although I did not know it then this would be the beginning of my ecological education.

Living in Copenhagen, the reputed capital of pornography, I was confronted with a paradox: I had never felt so safe walking down the street as a woman alone. My daily interactions and general crime statistics made it quite plain that Danish society was simply less brutal and violent than any I had ever known. I sensed that the harm of pornography could not be posited in a simple causal fashion that took no account of the particular cultural context.

I returned to the United States in the fall of 1981 to find a much stronger antipornography movement and a feminist

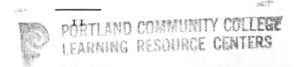

movement that was increasingly divided on the issue. I did not think pornography was harmless; I had no doubt that, for example, when pornographic pictures permeated a workplace it created a situation that was intolerable for the women working there. Pornography, in its dominant heterosexist form, makes women into things, propagating a vision of eroticism that denigrates women. Yet I found myself bothered by an emergent feminist stance that pornography was the root cause of women's oppression. This view did not fit very well with what I had felt in Denmark. I was drawn, instead, to the dense yet compelling ideas that had just been articulated by Susan Griffin in *Pornography and Silence: Culture's Revenge against Nature.* Griffin argued that pornography in the West was the expression of the culture's delusion that it could control nature. Under this interpretation, the debasement and humiliation of women is viewed in the context of the pornographic fear and hatred of the body and nature.[2] I did not yet fully grasp Griffin's larger message that healthy selves accept death and accept that "we are sometimes quite powerless before the powerful circumstances of this earth," but I was beginning to have serious doubts about efforts to control pornography through the power of the state.[3]

While I had already begun to question the strategy of using the state in the fight against pornography, I had not seriously questioned the more general feminist premise of drawing on the power of the state to expand women's political possibilities. Like so many women of my generation I had long assumed that the assertion of women's right regarding our bodies was the most radical; without this most basic form of control our hope for freeing ourselves from patriarchy was for naught. It was in the context of these reflections about strategy and theory that I began the journey which has generated the questions of this book.

Reading the first volume of Michel Foucault's *The History of Sexuality* and the interviews and essays in the collection *Power/Knowledge* with a friend was an occasion to ponder the self-evident truths of feminism as we knew it. We reflected on the meaning of control, why contemporary peoples seemed so hungry for it, and whether contemporary feminism's basic slogan regarding women's right to control their bodies was complicitous in what Foucault called "the deployment of sexuality." Rather than a mark of freedom, we began to worry that the focus on controlling our bodies, and the feminist effort to discover our true sexuality might serve to strengthen the underlying assumptions of the scientific experts, media monopolists, and pornographers who equated pleasure with sex. Had our own feminist rhetoric become yet another mechanism for conflating a woman's self with sexuality, effectively limiting rather than expanding our awareness of available pleasures?

Foucault enabled us to understand that these problems of language were of a more general political and psychological nature as well. No amount of petitioning the state for enhanced individual "autonomy" or control, necessary though it might be in certain instances, could provide a way of transforming a liberal political culture in which individuality was understood as being only realizable in the realm of the private. We were groping for new languages capable of addressing the great problems of desire and agency that did not center on mastery or monolithic identity. Given the stridency of the feminist debates concerning pleasure and sexuality, Foucault offered insights about the historical construction of self, sexuality, and desire that seemed a way to move beyond Freudian discussions of orgasm and mother.

This initial questioning of feminist language had occurred in a small, conservative Midwestern college town where the population was almost completely white and alternative politics nonexistent. From there I moved to Southern California. In Los Angeles, the contours of consumer culture are perhaps starker than any place on the planet. In this strange place the clash between the deadly poisons of our "lifestyle" and the well-being of the fragile ecosystems that make this standard of living possible is especially vivid. Immense shopping malls spread over acres of previously fertile orange groves, planted in a sandy desert whose existence was dependent on water sluiced from hundreds of miles away, destroying one of the worlds most magnificent fresh water lakes. Billions of dollars are spent building streets, highways, and alleys, while engineers have created a machine which can tear up the asphalt and mulch the pavement, turning it back into what they claim is fertile soil.

Climbing in the rugged Santa Monica Mountains one morning, I found myself resting at a spot where I could see the vast panorama of the basin that held Los Angeles. With its towers engulfed by smog that made the San Gabriel mountains barely visible in the background, I felt I could almost touch the contradictory nature of this place. Yes, there was the homogenized world of plastic people, food, mindless entertainment, and the faceless weapons industry. At the same time, there were also glimpses of people eating organically grown food, hiking through snow-covered mountains and walking on a sunny beach in the same day, and enjoying connections with friends, family, and the earth that sustains all. In Los Angeles, I found friends and artists who chose to call the earth "she," many whose visionary imaginations were fueled by the idea of archaic Goddess-revering societies or the earth-based spiritual practices of many indigenous peoples. Antinuclear activists ceaselessly organized against the weapons industry and the construction of atomic power plants. Direct action politics was always on the agenda for any number of causes. Poor women of color in the inner city collectively stopped the construction of a waste incinerator in their neighborhood, their action temporarily dissolving an often unrecognized but all too real antagonism between social justice and ecological well-being in the United States.[4]

It was in this context that I initially learned of Petra Kelly and the West German Greens. In June of 1984 as Los Angeles's alternative community held a counter celebration to the hoopla of the Summer Olympics, I chanced on a group of activists and writers who were struggling to figure out what Green politics could mean on this side of the Atlantic. I discovered the beginnings of a vocabulary with which I could make some sense of what I had been experiencing. The emergent Greens who had recently won governmental posts in West Germany were opening new political horizons.[5] In calling themselves "the fundamental alternative" the Greens asked if there were other ways to achieve the ideals of the French and American revolutions—liberty, equality, solidarity—without resorting to the dated and debilitating forms of liberal politics. The Greens had come to global attention by entering a national parliament. Yet their notion of "think globally, act locally," and their mocking of the staid procedures of the parliamentary body they had just entered spoke vividly to the limits of nation-state politics. I was intrigued by this self-declared "anti-party party" that offered an innovative program based on ecological wisdom, non-violence, decentralism, and social justice, and joined in the effort to create a Green presence in the United States. As I began a study of the burgeoning surrogacy industry in Los Angeles I learned that the women of the West German Greens, who gravitated toward the term "ecofeminist," also shared my concerns about the acclaimed new reproductive technologies. While these new reproductive technologies offer some women hope and happiness, their focus on the manipulation of women's bodies to bear children at any physical and monetary cost, intensifies some of the worst features of the materialistic and technologized contemporary world.

In Los Angeles, with my growing sense of an ecological self and my interest in conceiving a new baby, I reentered the world of gynecological care which had been radically reconfigured since my experiences almost two decades before. In 1985, I could readily get advice from women doctors and new genetic counselors who were primarily women, but my positive feelings faded as I faced the harrowing choices the new technologies of more risk-free pregnancy offered. The opportunity to say yes to abortion when an obscure blood test said something was wrong with a baby that was fervently desired seemed mixed at best. The women I met, whether doctors or counselors, were credentialed as experts by a society obsessed with technological manipulation and fearful of the uncertainties of living. One newly trained woman doctor recommended a hysterectomy for my diagnosed fibroids, another focused more on the possibilities of carrying a pregnancy to term in such a "sick" condition and offered data about the local hospital's ability to rescue babies from the womb at ever earlier ages, while an older nurse midwife gently directed me to an older male physician who still used his hands in assessing the course of pregnancies and deliveries.

Living in the Pacific Northwest for the past five years, adjacent to the last remnant of temperate rain forest in North America, I have come to a fuller appreciation of the complicated webs of connection that shape my health and that of my young daughter, who I miraculously gave birth to several days after my forty-third birthday and too many years on the I.U.D. In this place that is now my home, I have learned that the intricate ecosystem that is the forest sustains a vast array of life. I now know that forests are not merely a collection of trees, and I have also seen what happens when the absence of this ecological wisdom shapes an entire economy and way of life. Oregon's forests are the basis of a powerful timber industry, a crucial component of the state economy. Driving on any highway one can easily see the results of industrial forestry whose practice of clearcutting many liken to rape. Clearly, the management practices of the huge "forest resources" conglomerates do not contain the basic idea common to most indigenous cultures—that one should treat the forest's abundance as a gift.[6] In Oregon the riches of the highly complex ancient forest have been systematically depleted by the corporate conglomerates. And contemporary workers, who understandably prefer laboring in the forest to the dole or assembly line, have lost the ability to understand the forest as a living ecosystem and a place for a viable livelihood.

My questioning of my surroundings has been shaped by an emergent ecofeminist discourse that brings into view parallels between the abuse of the forests and the soil and the abuse of women. Learning and arguing with a friend who is not focused on exploring this connection but readily hears the wailing of the majestic Douglas firs that inhabit this place, I have begun to grasp the awareness that grows from being rooted to a particular place. My friend knows the streets of Manhattan as I do, yet she has permitted herself to cultivate faculties that open her to the spirit here. Her intense love of the forest, her atunement to the most subtle details of Oregon's habitats and their nuances of change, gives me a glimpse of the erotics of place and community. I have come to a greater appreciation of the need for humility and the importance of knowing through a variety of senses. Yet I sometimes worry that I still mostly grasp these ecological truths as if they were the missing elements in an intellectual puzzle. My own struggle to recreate myself and find an appropriate politics for reclaiming the earth for all beings is still very much in process.

Grappling with the manifold ways that ecological sensibilities can change the feminist politics of women's bodies, in the spring of 1989 I journeyed to a conference in Comilla, a small town in rural Bangladesh. There, women from across the globe had gathered to report on the state of women's reproductive health and the threats of new reproductive technologies and genetic engineering. These women were not focused on the reputed problems associated with crowded living conditions. If that were the focus of their concern they might have gathered in densely settled countries such as Holland or Japan. Rather they were impassioned about the way in which reproductive technologies were being marketed as the solution to the poverty of the South. Here in this nation that has become the modern symbol of the horrors of "overpopulation," the distinction between the new reproductive technologies designed to facilitate conception and birth and the older birth control technologies designed to prevent conception was dissolved. Indeed, at this conference the abuses of in-vitro fertilization and other out of body conception processes competed for attention with the abuses of modern contraception that was the focus of concern for health activists from the South. It was here, in the midst of a debate between those who called for more stringent guidelines to insure that the testing of new contraceptives did not abuse women and those who insisted at any form of medical testing entailed the abuse of some women, inevitably women of color, I listened to Farida Akhter, a research field organizer for the local host organization who struggled to dissolve this impasse. Her call for attention to the imposition of Western constructions of sex and pleasure on local women begged the immediate question at hand—was there any resolution of such radically different worldviews regarding the possibilities of technology?. To me, though, she had hinted at other issues equally in need of investigation: Was it possible that the entire apparatus of modern contraception and reproductive planning was one of the crucial elements in the construction of heterosexual sex and desire? Was this apparatus integral to the deployment of white European notions of self and privacy across the globe? The effort by some conference participants to paint new reproductive technologies as but another assault in men's historic war against women's bodies was too simple. It was also necessary to recognize them as another effort to discipline and regulate human practices in the name of science and modernization; a burgeoning trend in the West that began in the seventeenth century. More-over, what was the link between these efforts to take charge of human life and efforts to demand constant productivity of the earth? I was drawn to some women activists who felt that an analysis of reproductive technologies needed to be tied to a critical perspective on growth and development more generally. They asked, as I did, what were the long-term cultural and ecological consequences of medical and agricultural technologies that were reshaping fertility in its many manifestations? I knew I would have to return to this complicated region for a more extended stay.

Recently I was fortunate enough to be able to live for over half the year in a bustling modern city in the Western Ghats of India. In this place the British called "Poona," now renamed Pune, the intersection of so many different modes of existence has ruptured the organization of space. One regularly took one's life in hand when crossing streets traversed by pedestrians, careening motor scooters, trucks and cars whose horns were usually blaring, bicyclists, and lumbering cows and bullock carts. As I listened and probed and visited remote villages struggling to maintain liveli-hoods and local practices against the onslaught of "progress" and its consumer pleasures, I knew there was no sure or simple response to the way in which late capitalist society was simultaneously homogenizing and ravaging the ecosystemic and cultural strengths of the planet. Poised against the West's overconsumption of the planet's riches the very framing of the environmental question as one of population versus resources seemed increasingly obtuse and hollow. Yet as I noticed who spoke the language of popula-tion control—the government bureaucrats, international aid donors, family planners, proud owners of spanking new condominiums, and tourists seeking to capture their exotic adventure with the right snapshot—and those who did not—village women who worked the soil, but no longer controlled the seeds they used for planting; the women health worker who regularly threw government supplied I.U.D.'s and birth control pills in the closet, while agitating for access to basic hospital care for the women she valiantly sought to serve and some regulation of the amniocentesis centers catering to women desperate to have male children; the lower caste servants who carried garbage and lovingly bathed the children of Brahmin employers who literally could not hear these women's words; and the poets, singers, and dancers who invited willing listeners "to listen to the wind from the South"—I knew it would not be easy to pierce the complicated layers of venality, history and reductive science that produced this language.

TODAY, THE MODE OF INSTRUMENTAL RATIONALITY, "THE notion that the rational mind could overcome the limitations of the body and nature within this world,"[7] has spread across the globe and threatens the survival of life itself. Women and children of the South have been the most victimized by the environmental degradation that accompanies instrumental plans and rational schemes to upgrade the bodies, soils, and waters of peoples whose practices do not conform to the needs of global capitalism. Feminist activists across the globe were the first to call attention to the gender dimensions of our contemporary environmental predicament, that is, the fact that women (and their children) disproportionately suffer when forests, land, water, animals, and the newest elements of nature—chemical toxins—are used as if there were to be no future generations. But feminist discourse in the West has not kept pace with the grass-roots activities of women around the world who are naming the linkages between the well-being of women's bodies and the integrity of the earth. My contention is that the Western discourse of reproduction and sexuality, focused so centrally on ideas of regulation and control, has made it difficult for many women in the West to see why the ecological activity of women must be considered integral to the feminist project.

I want to restate my concern regarding Western feminism in its boldest terms. My concern is that much of the discourse of women's liberation reinforces the will toward technological mastery in the modern West, a will to mastery which is at bottom antiecological. The paradox is that in the process of challenging women's exclusion from the "we" of history, feminist discourse has produced further support for patriarchal civilization's disdain of the human body and life's complicated cycles of birth, renewal, and withering.

To illuminate this paradox in this book, I interrogate the contemporary feminist tenet that a woman's freedom lies in the right to gain control over her body and sexuality, that women's control over reproduction is foundational. My focus is less on the complex of issues surrounding a "rights"-based politics—though this will come up in the course of investigation—than on the practices, values, and understandings of self and world embedded in and produced by a modern ideology of technological and scientific control. The defensive positions in which mainstream United States feminist groups such as the National Organization for Women and the National Abortion Rights Action League have often found themselves with respect to abortion, the confusion over the meaning of women's legal right to remain unsterilized while working in toxic workplaces, and the profound divisions among women across the globe over the "promise" of the new reproductive technologies are just a few indications of the problems that arise from modern feminism's reliance on the language of control of the body and sexuality.

I want to make clear that I am not questioning the basic feminist insistence that men have long controlled women in a variety of damaging ways. They have, and it is right for women to resist all such abuses of power. But at the same time, we must ask ourselves what phrases like "Our Bodies, Ourselves," "Woman's Body, Woman's Right," and "Sexuality is to feminism, what work is to marxism, that which is most one's own yet most taken away" really mean.[8] What understanding of self, community and world do these slogans contain? What vision is this feminist language imbued with? Does it effectively challenge the multicentered nature of contemporary practices of patriarchal power? And does it apply to the lives of women around the globe, when our awareness of the differences in women's situations makes it perilous to even speak of the category of "women"?

The background to the framing of control as women's liberation lies in the historical emergence of feminism out of liberalism as Mary Wollstonecraft and others critiqued yet embraced Enlightenment thinkers in the eighteenth century. The subsequent development of women's movements over the course of the nineteenth and twentieth centuries engaged different revolutionary and reform movements of their day. The nineteenth century's prevailing ideologies of Marxism and liberalism heavily shaped the contours and debates of feminism. Despite important philosophical differences between Marxism and liberalism, both ideologies took up the Enlightenment's uncritical acceptance of science and reason as the sole means for discovering truth and knowledge. Marxism's challenge to the economic rationality of the dominant bourgeois class, important as it was and still is in questioning the commoditization of the world, nonetheless still readily accepted the bourgeois class's notion of progress through the exercise of scientific control. Although many radical feminists in the West self-consciously rejected Marxism, modern feminism, in all its major strains, wholly emulated Marxism's utopian vision of seizing control, in this case of reproduction.

Prefigured by Charlotte Perkins Gilman's theoretical *Women and Economics* and utopian *Herland* at the opening of the twentieth century, contemporary feminist theorists and novelists have engaged in various efforts to assess why women have not had control over reproduction and sexuality and to imagine what women's control of reproduction would entail.[9] For example, the political scientist Rosalind Petchesky, in a compelling theoretical effort to ground women's reproductive freedom in the principle of controlling our bodies, traces the liberal origins of this notion to the Puritan revolution in seventeenth century England. Petchesky contends that the original notion of "'property in one's person' was not only an assertion of individualism in an abstract sense but had a particular radical edge that rejected the commodification of bodies through an emergent labor market."[10] Petchesky's contention that radicals cannot afford to blithely dismiss all liberal ideas is one I surely agree with. At the same time it is essential to look closely at the contemporary situation. Today's market is fully global, and whole cultures are manipulated by the enticements of ever greater choice and control. Scientific experts splice living persons down to their genes, persons argue for the right to sell their body parts, and hope and desire is inextricably bound up in sex and consumption. As the late Linda Singer astutely observed, "late capitalism has largely succeeded in establishing the articulation of needs and desires along two basic axes—genital gratification and satisfaction through consumption."[11] In this context we need to ask ourselves whether the discourse of property in one's person is adequate for challenging dominant power relations.

In thinking about these difficult issues, we will do well to take into account both grassroots feminist activists' ecological work and Foucault's theoretical observations about the operation of contemporary "power/knowledge." Though these perspectives are situated very differently, each remind us of the limits of human agency and calls into question conventional feminist and environmental discourse. Foucault might ask of feminism—be it in its liberal, radical, or socialist form—whether the notion of women gaining control over their bodies subverts or reinforces prevailing constructions of subjectivity and sexuality. Ecological activists, in their emphasis on webs of connection and social justice, remind us that bodies cannot exist apart from the earth, that diversity is what sustains life. From each perspective we might ask whether the dominant strategy for freeing women reinforces or subverts the standardization and exploitation of the cultural textures and biological riches requisite to any civilization. Each asks whether greater scientific and bureaucratic management of life truly enhances democratic politics.

My contention is that the concept of fertility is helpful for opening up and reframing contemporary feminist and environmental political discussions. An ancient term for the regenerative capacities of all life, today we find most aspects of fertility rudely commodified, mechanized, and scientized. The evocative term fertility is too easily abandoned by feminists because of its resonance of patriarchy.[12] But by allowing scientists, bureaucrats, and the market to determine the meaning of fertility, we have relinquished a central concept for understanding the embodied, cyclical nature of human existence. It is my hope that this book's approach to fertility—in which I include the productive capacities of women's bodies and the soil as well as the creative imagination of our minds—will demonstrate the frailty of resisting patriarchal control over women through reliance on the words and ideas of the master. The evidence is beginning to accumulate that neither our bodies, minds, hearts, nor the living earth are nourished by the dominant language of control. In contrast to this language which is ceaseless in its efforts to mold and manipulate, the more ancient language of fertility does not insist on constant productivity.

Since Thomas Malthus's opening of the modern discussion of human fertility in England in 1798, discourses of fertility control have been inseparable from the maintenance of gender, class, and racial hierarchies.[13] In the contemporary world these hierarchies have become especially complicated. On the one hand are the eugenic possibilities of new reproductive technologies, coupled with new calls for "population control" in nations of the South that are said to be using too many resources. And on the other hand are the ways in which the labor of third world women and men has been integrated into the global market and the ways in which the genetic diversity of the South's soil is being mined by biotech conglomerates. This disciplining of bodies and engineering of seeds in the nations of the South has been a crucial element in allowing peoples of the North to maintain their way of life and the dream that the natural world can be mastered and controlled.

Nowhere is this more evident than in what this book calls modern fertility politics. Ancient anti-woman dreams of fleeing the curse of the body that are so vividly marked in the tale of the Garden of Eden have been reshaped by modern techniques of power that operate less through corporeal punishment and religious thou shalt nots, and more through surveillance, enticement, and the norms of the human sciences. Gradually over the course of the last three hundred years, dreams of "food without sweat," "sex without consequences," and "children without turmoil," reactions to the cruel curses that God dealt Adam and Eve, have come to seem tantalizingly within our reach. Paradoxically, the closer to realization these dreams of freedom appear, the more effective they become as methods of control and discipline, coming to shape and penetrate almost every aspect of our consciousness. With the development of the capitalist industrial order permitting vast numbers of women and men to eat without working with soil or water, our lives became marked by manmade clocks and the truths of scientific experts. As this industrial and scientific order more fully encompassed the globe in the twentieth century, pulling women of all classes and all races into it, the dreams of sex without consequences and children without turmoil also appeared capable of realization. Today the effects of these dreams are not only found in our individual psyches, bedrooms, and doctors' offices, but in an array of educational, social service and development offices endeavoring to ever more fully integrate women into a planetary industrial/ consumer culture.

Throughout this book the politics of fertility—from the development of birth control movements in the United States and the state's involvement in family planning to the commodification and standardization of human procreation and food production across the globe—provides a concrete, theoretically rich touchstone for examining both the difficulties of feminism's dominant position regarding women's bodies and the environmental movement's dominant position regarding the deleterious impact of human numbers.

This book is divided into five main sections. The following chapter, "Bodies, Sex, and Feminist Politics: Echoes of Anger and Celebration," explains Foucault's relevance to the ecofeminist investigation of this book. The chapter suggests that the future promise of feminism is dependent on its ability to supplant the forms of rationality and agency that created the very possibility of feminism. In contrast to the dominant form of feminism, which shares our larger culture's anger at our dependence on the earth, I trace the emergence of a mode of politics that is more prone to celebrate these dependencies and to use languages that evoke a fuller range of our senses, emotions, intellect, and imagination. I consider why the discourses of celebration that speak of humility and limits to human power may be particularly appropriate in meeting the challenges of the contemporary era.

Chapter 3, "Sex without Consequences: From Sexual Freedom to the Sexuated Body," deals with debates about contraception, sexual pleasure, and motherhood as they emerged in the mid-nineteenth century United States, paying particular attention to the twentieth-century development of the state's involvement in family planning and contemporary debates about teenage sexuality and abortion. My argument is that until we see the complicated ways in which our pre-occupation with sex is susceptible to control through bureaucratic and scientific expertise, our health and sense of pleasure will be undermined, our politics will remain stag-nant, and our hope of a more inclusive democratic politics will remain an empty pipedream.

Chapter 4, "Children without Turmoil: From Sex with-out Reproduction to Reproduction without Sex," moves from a discussion of traditional family planning to the new reproductive technologies, such as extrahuman fertilization and genetic screening, that are said to offer even greater amounts of control and choice. I examine the debates among feminists regarding these newest reproductive technologies, highlighting the contradictions contemporary feminism increasingly encounters in its effort to ground women's free-dom in control of the body. The routinization of genetic screening technologies, based on the goal of alleviating pain and suffering, advances a standardization of human life, creating threats to the dignity and well-being of women and persons with disabilities, and to human life itself. The con-temporary focus on the threats that hide within our bodies enables us to look away from the threats to planetary life that our toxic system of production has produced.

Chapter 5, "Food without Sweat: From Abundance for All to the Poisoning of the Planet," shifts from the normal-ization and industrialization of human bodies to an exami-nation of how we have harnessed the earth's riches. I exam-ine how an industrial model of food production was built. Following World Wars I and II this model of growth was transferred to postcolonial nations through the project of development. I focus on the deterioration of the earth's capacities for renewal that accompanied these development efforts, paying particular attention to how ecological degradation had a negative impact on women's sustenance activities. It is particularly in this area that the convergence of feminism and ecology opens up new questions. Where both reform and radical environmental movements alike have often seen the problems of postcolonial nations in terms of "too many people," looking at the issue of sustainability through the eyes of women forces us to confront what population control has meant for women's lives. We can probe further by asking whether institutionalized family planning with its norm of the small nuclear consumer household actually disguises the mechanisms by which a global consumer society is produced. This refocusing asks us to recast the population question from one which focuses on the breeding and backwardness of the "other" to a question of the overconsumption in the developed world.

Chapter 6, "Our Bodies, Our Earth: The Politics of Renewal, Restructuring, and Re-evolution," does not argue for sex *with* consequences, children *with* turmoil, or food *with* sweat, but rather for a new formulation of our relationship to our bodies and the earth that does not entail binary oppositions. This chapter examines some of the alternatives to the ethic of control that are now being rediscovered and created around the globe by the individuals and groups that form the new constellation of ecofeminist/Green movements. Typically these groups link the well-being of women's and men's bodies with the well-being of the earth, opening up new possibilities for living with, rather than against, the natural world. This politics of renewal, which is strikingly anarchist in practice, is contrasted with the other major contemporary effort to save the earth, the politics of restructuring that is promoted by large nongovernmental environmental organizations, trans-national corporations, and international agencies. Despite the fact that this latter politics talks the language of limits, it does not recognize the virtues of humility, and instead seeks to secure the earth's well-being through highly elaborated forms of management and control. The emergent ecofeminist politics of re-evolution holds the possibility of reawakening our sense of our species being, perhaps opening up a democratic politics that can transform modern politics itself.

The book concludes with an afterword, "Coming to Rest." There I summarize the Jewish concept of Shabbat (Sabbath) and its possibilities for providing an alternative way of thinking about our technical civilization.

It is my hope that this book's ecofeminist approach to the subject of fertility will bring a fresh, nonbureaucratic, and caring perspective to the much debated issues of contraceptives for teens, abortion, new reproductive technologies, population control, and development. My goal is not so much to provide specific answers (i.e., policies), but to question established modes of thinking in order to illuminate the social movements whose resistance to the logic of control are essential to the challenges we all face.

My criticisms of feminist strategies may appear harsh, but they are not intended as support for any of the assorted arguments announcing the arrival of postfeminism. As I will demonstrate, some of the most imaginative and morally cogent alternatives to the dominant model of growth are being articulated within feminism. As Western feminism is challenged by the new social movements of post-colonial societies, the creativity unleashed by these complicated interactions bodes well for both feminism and the planet. The critique I make of the feminist movement, of which I am a part, is not for the purpose of assigning errors and failures but to discern paths for reconstruction.

The ecological visions that are currently being etched out across the globe often oppose women's reputed capacity to heal to men's destructiveness in a way that assumes an essential connection between women and "the natural." I am wary of these arguments claiming that women are closer to nature, however, and I endorse the questioning of this presumption. My own radically different experiences of pregnancy and birth make it very clear to me that women's experiences of their birthing bodies do not "naturally" translate into an understanding of specific truths about the world. Whatever knowledge a woman may gain from pregnancy is fully mediated by her understandings of self, aging, and the world. At the same time, though, I believe it is necessary to reflect on what else is included in much of the antiessentialist critique. A viewpoint that eschews any aspect of essentialism may carry a nihilism and/or arrogance that is antithetical to ecological sensibilities. In focusing on essentialist assumptions regarding women and men, it is possible to miss the reconstructive potential brought into play by contemporary peace and ecological movements. Because their tactics are often geared to exposing the limits of human mastery and control, these movements often destabilize and puncture prevailing constructions of gender and the human. At issue is the question of how we may create images and visions of living with our bodies and the earth in a world where our earthly existence is systemically hidden and denied.

From an ecofeminist perspective, the breakdown of Western metaphysics, or the "postmodern condition," contains within it much more reason for hope than many of its academic apostles would lead one to believe. The loss of historical verities concerning values, cultures, and persons allows all of us to imagine the world anew. The imagination of an invigorated, caring democratic politics that offers a fitting alternative to the engulfing arm of the contemporary state will demand vast amounts of will and love on the part of both women and men. For guidance we have such prefigurative healers as Walt Whitman, Dorothy Day, and Mahatma Gandhi, the wisdom and sciences of contemporary indigenous peoples and the visions of an entire generation of creative storytellers, artists, and witches, who in the process of invoking spirit and recovering mythic images of forgotten goddesses are representing a nonpatriarchal cosmos.

BODIES, SEX, AND FEMINIST POLITICS: ECHOES OF ANGER AND CELEBRATION

The 'control of nature' is a phrase conceived in arrogance, born of the Neanderthal age of biology and philosophy.

RACHEL CARSON,
The Silent Spring

Without rage, any discussion of a feminist world would be tooth-less, blind to concrete pain and terror. And without hope, there would be no movement toward another way of being. Hope springs from a strong belief that all creation is very much intertwined, that all life is sacred. A feminist world would recognize our bonds with one another and the trees and the birds and the animals. With that recognition would come a celebration of our differences.

ADELE SMITH-PENNIMAN,
"Envisioning A Feminist World," Woman of Power

ON THE SIMPLEST OF LEVELS, THE ANCIENT STORY of Echo and Narcissus helps to remind us that in patriarchal culture women have limited capacity for speech. The fate of Echo was that she could only be a listener, she could only reiterate what had already been said. Echo's plight can make us mindful of the difficulties contemporary feminism faces in struggling to oppose patriarchal control while still speaking the language of patriarchal discourse. Echo's unrequited love for Narcissus, who was poisoned by drinking his own image, also warns of the danger of becoming entrapped by our initial ideals and images. Narcissus's seduction by his own image both underscores the fatal consequences of visions that have become stagnant and the danger of overreliance on our visual sense.[1]

The dilemma of feminism in the late twentieth century is that its promise of political, cultural, and even spiritual renewal depends upon its ability to supplant the modern forms of rationality and agency which created the very possibility of women's social and political movements in the West. Mary Wollstonecraft's eighteenth century citizen/mother who exercised the same reasons as Rousseau's male citizen inspired women to action in the Enlightenment age of reason, and her challenges to masculine authority have proven inspirational to women's movements to this day. In the twentieth century, the compelling credo of women's liberation, perhaps most powerfully articulated in Simone de Beauvoir's *The Second Sex,* was invaluable in exposing the extensiveness of patriarchal domination and in constructing a female subject willing to attack it. For de Beauvoir, who admired reason as Wollstonecraft did, women's freedom was integrally related to the technological regulation of fertility. Pregnancy, essentially slavery in de Beauvoir's view, alienated a woman from herself, making it difficult for her to be the agent of her own destiny and engage in the project-making that could lead to "transcendence."[2] In distinct contrast to Wollstonecraft and nineteenth century women's activists, de Beauvoir cast childbearing and domestic work as activities that involved mere repetition, or "immanence," and thus were to be avoided.

In the United States, de Beauvoir's text was taken up by young women in the 1960s and was one of the important catalysts that led these women to examine their own lives. As they began to explore how women's subordination was maintained within all the institutions of society—from the church and the workplace to the supposedly most private and intimate of places, the family—they began to assert their resistance to the patriarchal logic that justified men's control over women. During this tumultuous period pamphlets such as "The myth of the vaginal orgasm" were circulated through informal networks, and women began to explore their sexual desires, which they argued had never been allowed free expression within the confines of patriarchy. Many women who had experienced sexual abuse by their male comrades set about organizing a resistance movement. Modern feminist politics which named patriarchal oppression in terms of the sexual came into its own.

Margaret Sanger had claimed in the early twentieth century that a woman's right to own and control her body was the fundamental route to freedom. For this new wave of feminists, Sanger's position resonated in a way that it had not for her contemporaries in the 1910s and 1920s. As Juliet Mitchell observed in 1971, "The sexual exploitation of women and their enforced submission within a society committed—when it feels like it—to the naturalness of their reproductive role, has caused the (women's) movement to develop the notion of the 'control of one's body.'"[3] Casting "women's liberation" in the language of control of the body and sexuality became a powerful tool for mobilizing women. This rhetoric spoke on the one hand to women's desire for sexual pleasure, and on the other hand to women's fears of abuse by men. For contemporary feminism, the right to control one's body and sexuality came to be seen as the most radical demand women could make. Women argued that if such control were realized, women—indeed, all of society—would experience the most profound revolution ever.

But more than two decades later we can discern some of the problems associated with our reliance on this language. In my view, mainstream feminism in the West has become in some ways trapped and stalemated by its once emancipatory vision that women's freedom resided in gaining control over our bodies and sexuality. Intense battles over lesbianism, sadomasochism, bisexuality, pornography, prostitution, contemporary sex industries, and the surrogacy industry have deeply divided Western feminists. The ideology of control has gradually narrowed our feminist visions into minute investigations of "sexuality," forcing us into internal debates and political stalemates. Accepting the dominant culture's definition of sexuality as identity, we have participated in a "wild-goose chase in pursuit of a true nature, an authentic self that lies, we are told, beneath our repressed sexuality."[4] Much is surely at stake when definitions of identity are at issue; however, by placing sexuality at the core of our search, it often seems that we have produced as many problems as we have resolved.

In the United States the continuing battle over abortion,

which painfully pits women against women, is perhaps the most visible political manifestation of the difficulty into which the search for control and the language of owning our bodies has taken us. Western feminism's focus on maintaining access to abortion in the face of challenges by religious and conservative forces has in many ways stifled feminist politics. Most obviously the political energies involved in defending the issue of legal access has made it difficult to elaborate a fuller platform of what we hope to achieve. But the more crucial issue, in terms of my concerns in this book, is the totalizing and homogenizing effects of the language feminists use to defend abortion. First there is the problem of defining sexuality as our core identity that I will develop more fully shortly. More specifically, with respect to abortion, there are unfortunate consequences of talking about abortion so as to suggest that women have sex only with men. Second, this dominant discourse of gaining control has made it difficult for feminist to appreciate the situations of women, most typically women at the bottom of racial and class hierarchies, for whom the greater access to techniques for curtailing fertility is often not the result of freedoms they have struggled for, but the effect of greater state intrusion into their lives.

Our use of the language of gaining control over our bodies and sexuality has certainly provided a basis of unity for Western feminism. At the same time it has made it difficult to respond to the sterilization and contraceptive abuses of women across the globe. Thus, for example, reform-minded feminist groups in the United States have often opposed mandatory waiting periods for sterilization procedures, insisting on unencumbered access for the woman who would choose this procedure to curb her fertility.[5] For many Native American women, however, whose fertility signals disorder to welfare state officials and medical personnel, sterilizations and hysterectomies are procedures they want protection from. As Az Carmen observes, "The early 70's saw American Indian women faced with a frightening attempt by the U.S. government, at removing their ability to insure their existence as peoples; genocide through the sterilization of all Indian women of childbearing age receiving care at Indian Health Centers. If this had happened to a species of tree or animal the hue and cry that would have arisen would have been difficult to ignore, yet because it happened to Indian women little is even know of what was happening.[6]

Most recently some feminist reformers have agitated for making the recently legalized contraceptive implant—Norplant—more widely available, while other poorer women have had to employ the legal system to insist on their right to move about in the world *without* having this hormonal implant under their skin.[7] Since the mid seventies, a period when the right to abortion in the United States has been under attack, it has proven difficult to develop a political perspective that also encompasses the issue, in places across the globe, of *freedom from* coercive "family planning choices." The language of control over the body might be used to defend against state efforts to regulate the availability of abortion, but within in the realm of North-South relations, this language has provided yet another technique by which established authorities police women's lives. In the relatively near future, one can easily imagine that the enticement of the new reproductive technologies will cause battles among women that rival those over pornography and abortion in the recent past. And perhaps the grimmest reminder that transforming sexual relations may have minimal impact on women's lives is the emerging evidence that across the globe women and their children (as well as tribal peoples) constitute a greater proportion of the poor than ever before.[8]

Of course it is important to note that in recent years there has been considerable feminist reconsideration of the devaluation of women implicit in Simone de Beauvoir's formulation of freedom. Adrienne Rich in her pathbreaking

1976 text *Of Woman Born,* offered language that enabled women to experience their physicality as a resource, making the startling claim that it was necessary to distinguish between motherhood as an institutional construction of patriarchy and motherhood as experience.[9] In a dramatic refutation of de Beauvoir's statements on the bondage of maternity, one line of feminist thought—represented by such diverse thinkers as Nancy Hartsock, a North American feminist Marxist political scientist; Julia Kristeva, a French feminist psychoanalyst; Maria Mies, a German ecofeminist sociologist; and Sara Ruddick, a feminist peace activist, teacher, and writer based in New York City—contends that the rationality inscribed in the daily practices of mothers provides a standpoint for critiquing patriarchy and bringing about a more egalitarian society which does not rely on de Beauvoir's categories.[10] Hartsock, for example, in *Money, Sex, and Power,* contends that, "Generalizing the human possibilities present in the life activity of women to the social system as a whole would raise, for the first time in human history, the possibility of a fully human communi-ty."[11] Ruddick, in *Maternal Thinking,* argues that "Western conceptions of what it is to be reasonable are intertwined with a fear and resentment of birthing female bodies."[12] Expanding upon the intelligence of the complex and cre-ative activities of child-rearing, Ruddick suggests that "maternal thinking" may be the appropriate vehicle for transforming politics and the world.

Neither is this reconsidering purely a historical or theo-retical matter. A second issue of considerable practical con-cern to many women today, especially those who are approaching the end of their fertile years, is how to fulfill their desire to have children. In the contemporary world, this desire can be fulfilled through the choices afforded by the newest reproductive technologies. Women no longer need to be constrained by the structures of the patriarchal family or the aging of their bodies. They can employ the wonders of genetic screening, artificial insemination, in vitro fertilization or the transfer and flushing of embryos to realize their dreams of bearing perfect children. This dream of flawless progeny is fed by scientific experts who teach us that we are our genes, through and through.

I too have been fascinated by the seemingly endless permutations of familial relations produced by the new techniques shaping fertility and our bodies more generally. Yet whatever its particular expression, from the notion that abortion is the linchpin of women's freedom to the demand for greater access to in-vitro fertilization or prenatal testing, the formulation of freedom as bodily control in contemporary feminist politics often parallels the masculine will to mastery that feminist have so forcefully criticized. Western feminism shares the masculinist culture's vision of the body as an object that can be preserved and improved upon through technological prowess. It is, admittedly, a vision with considerable appeal in our contemporary world, but it also systematically ignores the highly complex ecological, cultural, and social webs that sustain all organic life.

Mainstream Western feminism is still heavily implicated in the separation of mind and body and body from earth that reigns in the West, rarely questioning the patriarchal and racist arrogance in which this language of control is embedded. We have forgotten the wisdom that was summed up so well centuries ago by Euripides: "A knowing mind that ignores its own limits has a very short span."[13] Deluding ourselves with myths of our own omnipotence and independence, we seek to mold the natural world to conform to our every desire, most especially sexual desire.

In the midst of the fierce political battles within modern feminism though, new visions of bodies are being etched out on the periphery of institutionalized feminism and institutionalized environmentalism in those places across the globe where respect for the earth's own designs is a given, where greater bureaucratic management and policing are scorned rather than applauded, and where women have had enough of population control and development schemes. We can observe the emergence of what might be termed "earth conscious" practices, which I term ecofeminist or simply Green; practices as diverse as direct action to expose established authority, song, blessings, witchcraft, art, poetry, and the shabirs, or ecological community "teach-ins," of India. Their creative blend of ritual, education, and politics warrants serious attention.

De Beauvoir made the crucial observation that patriarchal culture constructs both woman and nature as the "Other" to be crushed and exploited. Yet her admiration of masculine values and projects led her to promote the full integration of women in the very culture that had produced this oppositional dialectic. In contrast to de Beauvoir, ecofeminist and Green movements question values and practices that seek to obscure our embodied existence. Indeed, for many ecofeminists who invoke the circle of life with its rhythmic flows and energies, even stones are alive and are in fact often used as grounding and healing tools in a world that is understood as dismembered and deeply ill. From this perspective Echo's change into stone may be understood not as the final death knell, but as a transformation enabling contemporary women and men to reflectively pause, to slow down enough so as to be open to alternative modes of apprehending knowledge and divinity.

Ecofeminists do not flinch from naming and resisting abuses of power, but unlike more traditional resistance movements, their strategy of change generally does not insist on heightening existing conflicts. The metaphor of the web of life recurs in many forms in ecofeminist practice, from the wrapping of wool around bastions of militarism, to the entrapment of police motorcycles in yarn, to the hugging of trees by the Chipko women in India to prevent logging. Ecofeminist practices creatively resist institutionalized authority and its tendencies toward violence, while envisioning more sensuously connected, fluid, and embodied modes of being. The web metaphor may perhaps be understood as a sign of ecofeminism's willingness to struggle and to use demolition tactics, yet refuse to decimate its Other.

In the postmodern era, what were once held to be universal truths have been exposed as ideas constructed to legitimate hierarchy, and the possibility of serious social transformation seems to have evaporated. In response to these circumstances ecofeminism offers a different celebratory mode of knowledge production that may be particularly appropriate for the political and cultural challenges of this confusing period. The word celebrate suggests plurality and festivity. It is especially celebration's less widely used connotation of "plurality" or "multiplicity" that ecofeminist politics stresses. Scientific and market-based epistemologies that insist on ordering and disciplining difference surely dominate the globe today. But struggling against this regulation of difference are those who claim that diversity is a source of strength and unity. Taking a cue from the diversity that sustains healthy ecosystems, ecofeminist writers and activists around the globe articulate languages, songs, and practices that enable humans, with all their particularities, to celebrate the experience of being intertwined, to experience the common bonds that sustain life. Through their insistence on calling attention to the multitude of connections between a fertile Earth and the well-being of her many cultures and creatures, ecofeminists point to richer, more inclusive visions for feminism. An appreciation of fertility in all its manifestations is central to maintaining this celebratory politics.

In light of my bold promises for ecofeminist politics, I recognize the need to more fully identify this strain of feminism. This is not a simple task; the varieties of ecofeminist activities across the globe testify to the fact that this emergent constellations does not have a simple lineage. Though ecofeminist politics is not solely rooted in feminism, the roots of activism for many of its participants are feminist, and in the absence of contemporary feminist movements, this new form of politics would never have come to be. Still, I believe a critique of Western feminism's reliance on the language of control of the body and sexuality is needed. My critique derives in large part from concerns about how use of this language in the contemporary world reinforces a matrix of power that according to Michel Foucault has made "sex the explanation for everything."[14] Thus before turning to a fuller consideration of the relationship between feminism and ecofeminist politics, I want to briefly explain why I have found Foucault's investigations so helpful in illuminating the echoes of patriarchy within contemporary feminist discourse.

Although Western feminism broke from the New Left in the 1960s, declaring that "the sexual revolution is not our revolution," in practice feminism has had great difficulty developing a countervision to the idea that sexuality is in itself the means to liberation. Contemporary feminist politics in North America oscillates between the antiviolence positions of writer/activists such as Catharine MacKinnon and Andrea Dworkin, who see sex as acts of violence and rape, on the one had, and the writings of such writer/activists as Kate Roiphe, Ellen Willis, Barbara Ehrenreich, and Carole Vance, who insist on women's agency when it comes to sex, on the other.[15] But both kinds of visions are constrained by the confluence of science, sex, and power that marks the contemporary West and is rapidly penetrating the remaining cultures on the planet.

Michel Foucault's work points to contemporary culture's tendency to see sex as the measure of identity and instrument of truth. Indeed, for Foucault, the universal gendered facts and practices that we think of as "sexuality" are actually a recent historical phenomenon, having emerged in the eighteenth and nineteenth centuries as a consequence of discourses that directed the question of what we are to sex.

Toward the beginning of the eighteenth century, Foucault argues, power, understood as a network of noncentralized, mobile forces, induced a "deployment of sexuality" in a society where, though he makes no note of it, the apparatuses of modern reductionist science had already begun to render the earth into an inert machine.[16] For Foucault, "The deployment of sexuality has its reason for being, not in reproducing itself, but in proliferating, innovating, annexing, creating, and penetrating populations in an increasingly detailed way, and in controlling populations in an increasingly comprehensive way."[17] For Foucault, power is no longer vested only in the sovereign's "right of seizure" but is now also a "power bent on generating forces, making them grown, and ordering them."[18] This new form of productive power he sometimes calls "disciplinary power" and sometimes "biopower." The modern nation state permitted the concealment of the new "microcenters" of power—the welfare state offices, the human development research centers, the psychiatrists' and gynecologists' offices, the biologists' laboratories—which operate through the production, policing, self-surveillance, and labeling of human activities. These processes, he argues, lead to a "society of normalization," a society governed less by legal rights than by the authority of the human sciences.

In the nineteenth century, as this normalizing process gained ascendancy, the developing disciplines of medicine, education, and psychology focused their investigations on the human body, probing the secret it was said to harbor: sex. This confluence of science, sex, and power produced, and continues to produce, an intensified focus on sexuality.[19] Thus our selves become joined inextricably to our body, which in turn is experienced exclusively in terms of sex, creating what might be called the "sexuated body," a body situated in, satiated with, and standardized by genital sex. Paradoxically, in a society that sees privacy and sexual intimacy as the realm for the deepest expression of individuality, even bedroom "techniques" have been processed for us in mass marketed videotapes and books. This commodification of sex has had profound and baleful consequences for our understanding of the erotic, eviscerating our capacities for pleasure. In effect, the creation of the sexuated body diminished our abilities to explore the gratifications of solitude, community, and sensuous connections with the world around us.

Foucault does not particularly illuminate the effects of normalization of sex on the lives of women—the routinization of battery, sexual exploitation, harassment, and sexual abuse in contemporary society. These are some of the darkest by-products of what he has called the "technologies of sex." Such technologies include pornographic material available in magazines, on cable television, over telephones, in video games, and on computer networks; the marketing of escort services, sexual paraphernalia, vaginal deodorants, and products to hide menstrual bleeding; the pharmaceutical industry's ceaseless search for the perfect contraceptive; the promotion of sex manuals that cater to perfecting a myriad of sexual practices; the array of therapeutic techniques for discovering true sexual identity; and the invention of "outing" as a cry of protest. Feminism has clearly reacted against many of these technologies, as evidenced by demonstrations against the objectification of women's bodies and the continuing appeal of the antipornography movement. Yet feminism is also implicated in them: perhaps the clearest example is the early popularity among feminists of the sexologists Masters and Johnson, whose works have also been the gospels of *Playboy*. And more recently, Sherry Lansing, the head of Paramount Pictures, defended the film "Indecent Proposal," in which a woman accepts a billionaire's $1 million offer in exchange for a night in bed, as "the ultimate feminist statement" because the woman was "deciding what she wants to do with her body."[20]

In the West in the late twentieth century (where Germaine Greer aptly notes, "sex is the lubricant of the consumer economy"[21]), the relationship between feminism and ecofeminist politics is complicated.[22] In my effort to outline some of the problems the discourse of control and sexuality poses for feminism I have admittedly ignored differences within feminism. Socialist feminists might respond that they have always tried to link control of the body with the totality of women's freedom, insisting on a notion of reproductive rights that was not solely limited to abortion. Liberal feminists might argue that they focus on matters of equality and access without reducing their politics to sexual issues. Each faction might argue that the problems I have outlined pertain only to radical feminism. In emphasizing differences within feminism, however, the effects of feminist discourse on larger understandings of self and world tend to be obscured.

The ideological categorization of different feminisms made a good deal of descriptive sense in the initial phase of this second wave of feminism, when women struggled to see how their efforts advanced or contradicted traditional secular visions of political liberation. In the ensuing twenty years, however, the challenges to the unified subject and transcendental truth of Enlightenment reason and humanism—from feminists, poststructuralists and diverse contemporary oppositional movements—has been so thoroughgoing that the categories of liberal, socialist, or Marxist no longer provide much ground for differentiating various groups, linked as they all are to a general framework that assumes bounded selves who achieve progress through material and technical advances. Today, a focus on the varied ideological strains within feminism, all of which are linked to Enlightenment approaches to liberation, limits our vocabulary of social transformation. The Enlightenment view claims that healthy human selves necessarily experience clear boundaries from the surrounding world; that humans are distinctly different from animals; and that all the phenomena of society and the natural world are appropriate objects of human will and "rational" control. It is this intellectual lineage, with its tricky philosophical and practical issues regarding truth and agency that the various movements called ecofeminist and Green confront.

Ecofeminists insist that women can take their place as moral agents in the world without treating the world as if it existed merely for our taking. For ecofeminists not all forms of possible creative praxis are justified or beneficial.

This insistence that the Earth is a living entity that must be defended and exalted springs from a recognition of the toxic consequence of contemporary Western consciousness—that the Earth has been rendered into an "it." In the West, physical, sensuous, and emotional connections with the world have weakened as the deployment of sexuality and industrial modes of living have accelerated. Renaming the Earth "she" may recover a sense of the Earth as a living being, sustaining manifold forms of life, and of other cultures' understandings of the links between the cycles of the body and the cosmos. Under this interpretation, the invention of grounding rituals to facilitate earthly sensibilities is not frivolous play or naive romanticism. Indeed such reinventions are part of a necessary counterattack in the creation of new economies of bodies, pleasures, and space. Ecofeminists seek to create and acknowledge selves that do not become fearful or violent when boundaries between self and other become fluid.[23]

Though I advocate de-emphasizing differences within feminism, it is true that radical feminism has most often raised questions about the well-being of female bodies that are at the core of ecofeminism. In the last few decades, it was largely through the writings and activism of radical feminists that issues such as rape, lesbianism, mothering, eroticism, abuse of women, sexual harassment, or the relationship between woman's body and the Earth's body, were placed on the feminist agenda.[24] Interestingly, it was the radical feminist Shulamith Firestone, working within the terms of population control ideology that would be anathema to many of today's ecofeminists, who first raised the subject of feminism and ecology in 1970.[25] As the decade advanced it was through the deconstructive efforts of such different radical feminists as Adrienne Rich, Judy Grahn, Luisa Teish, Mary Daly, Susan Griffin, Sally Gearhart, Ynestra King, Ursula LeGuin, Audre Lorde, Alice Walker, Starhawk, and Paula Gunn Allen that the new terrain of thought regarding the body and the Earth was created, a terrain that began to expose the limits of control and the possibilities generated by greater openness to mystery and the unknown.[26]

I make this point not to demonstrate that radical feminism is the only true form of feminism, but to place ecofeminist politics in the United States within historical context. It is radical feminists who first began to question Western feminism's credo of "control over our bodies" and its echo of the dominant masculine logic of instrumental control. One way of understanding the development of ecofeminism is as an unfolding spiral or dialectic centered within radical feminist politics. It was within radical feminism that the language of the body and sexuality was most fully developed and it was also within radical feminism that the language of embodied bodies and pleasures gradually came to counterpose feminism's narcissistic tendencies.

Ecofeminist writers and activists see everything as interconnected and insistently reclaim the erotic while attending to the Earth's cycles of renewal and change. In this view, ecological understandings of human agency do not diminish human creativity. As the essayist Susan Griffin aptly puts it in writing alternatives to the arrogance of Western civilization, "But if you understand that your creative knowledge comes from participation in a knowledge larger than yourself you must somehow be humbled. You begin to sense your limitations as a single being."[27] The promise of ecofeminist politics derives from its awareness that these "limitations" can serve as a source of strength. This revaluation and promotion of the virtue of humility as an enabling force links ecofeminism with that strand of radical feminism that became the feminist peace and antinuclear movements in the late 1970s. The feminist claim that the "personal is political" was transformed into the claim "the local is global." The Women's Pentagon Actions in the United States, the encampment at Greenham Common in Great Britain and the women's peace camps, sit-ins, and demonstrations in North America, Western Europe, Japan, and the South Pacific creatively used chants, puppetry, ritual dances, and webs of wool to simultaneously expose militarism and technology gone amok, and to point to more connected ways of living.[28] One of the strengths of ecofeminist politics today is that it has inherited this important political history of radical feminism's peace politics.

Nonetheless, the question still remains as to how an Earth-conscious politics might flourish in a world that is currently governed by masculine values and in which there are no serious alternatives to capitalism. In my view, at least part of the answer lies in creating feminist language that does not echo the dominant culture's anger at our dependence on the Earth and its placement of the sacred in the skies. The claim that the desecration of the Earth is a result of a specifically masculine consciousness that devalues women's experiences originated within ecofeminist scholarship and activism. Women in both the North and South are pushing beneath the accepted literary, theological, and historical canons to revalue women's cultures and practices attuned to the phases of the moon, to reclaim goddess imagery, and to consider the possibility of prepatriarchal cosmologies that did not rely on a transcendental deity.[29] As Carolyn Merchant aptly notes, "Transcendence undermines the epistemological equality of the senses through its emphasis on the visual. Here truth is the light of God, knowing is seeing, and knowledge is illumination. Vision as the primary source of knowledge creates an observer distant from nature. Knowledge gained through the body by touch, smell and taste is degraded in favor of knowledge modeled on perspective.[30] Ecofeminist practice is intimately involved in contesting our dominant culture's epistemological and theological categories, using dance, chants, drumming rituals, and more to revive our senses and gain access to multiple forms of knowing and being.

This simultaneous opening up and de-centering of knowledge, the empowering sublimation of hubris and the re-opening of discussions of the sacred, permit a range of new utopian narratives. These stories, regardless of their "truth" as defined in Enlightenment terms that reject the non-visual, have been put forth by a variety of "responsible dreamers" across the planet.[31] Historian of science Donna Haraway, for example, avails herself of the fluidity and possibilities of postmodernism in the playful dreams of cyborgs. Haraway imagines that the breakdown of boundaries between contemporary humans, our technologies, and the "natural" opens the possibility of "earthly survival."[32] Philosopher Lorraine Code remaps the epistemic terrain of modern philosophy by proposing that an ecological model could shift inquiry away from our obsession with autonomy. For Code, "Ecologically rather than individualistically positioned, human beings are interdependent creatures, 'second persons' who rely on one another as much in knowledge as they do for other means of survival."[33] Archaeological and religion scholars have found hope of a more sustainable future in reconstructions of a goddess-worshiping past. These emergent goddess paradigms have often been labeled romantic, but in my view, such critiques reflect our patriarchal culture's incapacity to recognize the important epistemological, ontological, and political transformations these cosmologies intend. As the feminist legal scholar Drucilla Cornell aptly puts it,

We are never simply working that "is," because what is, is only "reachable" in metaphor, and therefore, in the traditional sense, not reachable. . . . The dreamer may be a visionary, but that does not mean that she sees any less well. . . . The necessary utopian moment in feminism lies precisely in our opening up the possibility for metaphoric transformation.[34]

Both the cyborg and the goddess stories provide important metaphors, suggesting a diverse array of practices—from organic farming, roof top gardening, community supported agriculture, and diets low on the food chain, to small dam projects, alternative forestry collectives, and holistic healing practices that attend to the phases of the moon—that counter the dominant world view of the body and earth as inert machines that are to be used and used up. These alternative practices offer the possibility of sustainability, social justice, and democratic empowerment. For ecofeminists of all ideological hues, the effectiveness of our protests against the ravages of technocratic growth is intimately related to our daily efforts to heal the earth.

Just as ecofeminist politics dos not have a single lineage within feminism, this emergent politics must also be understood within the context of various contemporary ecological movements, especially those that have attempted to learn from the wisdom of indigenous peoples. Individual groups within the worldwide Green movement surely differ in the specific issues and strategies they pursue. Indian grass-roots movements protest the construction of massive dam projects, saying no to the development schemes of both the state and the World Bank, while movements in the industrialized North are saying no to the use of bovine growth hormones in the dairy industry and animal experimentation in the cosmetics and medical research industries. Yet what joins them together under a Green umbrella is their questioning of the Western ideology of linear, secular progress and Western science's displacement of traditional healing and agricultural practices. This insistence on taking heed of marginalized knowledges as well as marginalized peoples is essential to the new ecological understanding of humans and the cosmos.

Women around the world, be they midwives, farmers, artists, or mothers, are an integral part of this challenge. Their daily activities in tending to the well-being of future generations provides them with a long-range vantage point from which they can readily assess the costs of quick-fix solutions. In the South, women are in the forefront of efforts to save the forests because their livelihood depends on balanced ecosystem rather than agricultural practices that weaken the soil and pollute the water. In the industrialized nations women are in the forefront of efforts to fight nuclear power and clean up toxic-dump sites. In both the South and North, from the Bhopal tragedy in India, where thousands were maimed by an "accident" in the production of pesticides to the "Bitter Fog" created along the coast of Oregon in the United States through the aerial bombardment of herbicides, the disruption of the cycles of species regeneration are made visible in women's bodies.[35] Spontaneous abortions and birth defects typically serve as early warning signals of the deadly cancers that man-made production of chemicals inevitably produce.

But women are refusing to be passive victims, taking their inspiration from women's actions around the globe, past and present. For example, the Chipko movement in India, where women embraced trees with their bodies to stop the felling of forests, has inspired many thousands of women. The Chipko women took their inspiration from the Bishnoi community where, three hundred years ago, women gave their lives to save the sacred Khejri trees.[36] Women in South Central Los Angeles who stopped the placement of a waste to energy incinerator that was touted as a source of clean jobs for their already devastated community took their inspiration from Rosa Parks and others who refused to move to the back of the bus a quarter of a century earlier. Women's leadership in fighting technological modernization raises troubling questions about the assertion of governmental elites and development experts that the manipulative feats of the "green revolution" have enhanced the Earth's fertility and enhanced the quality of life for rural peoples.

For the activist/writers Vandana Shiva, Maria Mies, Gail Omvedt, Bina Agarwal, Gabriele Dietrich, and Helena Norberg-Hodge, who paint devastating stories of what development of the Indian subcontinent has meant for women, their communities, and the Earth, development is more appropriately viewed as a form of "maldevelopment" that we may need to resist with a form of "counterdevelopment" or "antidevelopment."[37] The ideals of progress and development, embedded as they are within modern science and capitalist marketing schemes, emphasize men's domination over women and the Earth, while simultaneously displacing rural women's, tribal peoples', and indigenous cultures' traditional ecological and community building practices.

Ecological feminism's ties to both radical feminism and the emergent Green movement can be problematic. The call for feminists to extend their concerns to the survival of the planet may be viewed as upholding the patriarchal construction of the nurturing woman as inextricably bound to nature, thereby avoiding the persistent issues of men's everyday violence against women. In addition, ecofeminists' attention to ritual and celebration may be viewed as nostalgic, romantic, and diversionary by Green activists who insist that the urgency of the planet's destruction demands clear and precise political action. Certainly, the echo of patriarchy has undermined some ecological reconstructive efforts. Women have reported, for example, that some communities of recent years advocated the view that the best way to bring in the new world was to fill it with ecologically friendly children. Earth mothers were to contribute to this task by procreating whenever men were so inclined. So, too, have some who celebrate the ecstasy of joyful connection become irresponsible dreamers rather than mindful repairers. A culture of narcissism will not disappear by our wishing it so; we should harbor no illusions about the difficult changes we have faced and will continue to face.

But I also believe that focusing on the essentialist errors of ecofeminism too easily allows us to avoid the unsettling metaphysical or theological challenges that ecofeminist politics presents to the contemporary practices of modern science and politics.

We must not err as young Narcissus did. We can make grievous mistakes with sometimes fatal consequences when we rely too heavily on the detached "objectivity" of our visual sense. A recultivation of knowledge from the full range of our senses is integral to the ecofeminist project. We must also be more critical of the visual images that shape our understanding of environmental problems, asking ourselves how these images and the narratives that accompany them have come to inhabit our minds. I would concur here with the literary theorist Andrew Ross who calls for a Green cultural criticism that would attend both to "images of ecology" and the "ecology of images."[38] Thus rather than accept the story of the planet's imminent demise as it is played out in newspaper front page stories, magazine special features, and best-sellers, we must attend more closely to the assumptions about nature, time, and the methods of quantification that construct these apocalyptic, "end of nature" scenarios. These doomsday scenarios can readily support schemes that insist on remaining in the thrall of the very technology that in many ways produced our contemporary predicament.

We need instead to remember and invent languages and images that speak of the wonder and beauty of the cosmos rather than the control of populations and the management of resources. Fostering an ethics of awe in the face of the majesty of creation is the work of sacred texts like the

Hebrew Bible. An ethic of awe recognizes the limits of human reason, and that nature is not fully comprehensible and may be resistant to our designs. One might call this sensibility, which manifests itself in the concrete, compassionate ways individuals tend to the well-being of their families, their neighbors, their villages, their extended communities, and the bioregions in which they live, "ecofeminist," although the label is not essential. What is essential is the development of a politics and practice that includes: (1) new definitions of liberation which acknowledge our ties with the other creatures who inhabit the Earth and break down the boundaries between self and world; (2) new languages and rituals which honor diversity and in so doing strengthen democratic politics; (3) new ethics which both allow us to hear the varied voices of nature (including those of humans) and acknowledge the morality of letting things be.

Thus, ecofeminist politics is not merely a joining together of women's rights with environmentalism to make new demands against the state. Ecofeminism is also a challenge to all the categories we use to order our experience in the Wester World. It poses fundamental questions to our understandings of our bodies (we do not have to fear and control them), our sense of pleasure and the erotic (pleasure is not only derived from sex but also from community building and sensuous connections to a living earth), our perception of difference (diversity is to be cherished as a source of creativity, sustainability, and democratic empowerment rather than exploited and devalued through hierarchies of race, gender, and sexual orientation), our perception of knowledge (truth is derived from all the senses rather than an exclusive reliance on the abstractions and quantifications of the visual), home (our home is the Earth which we share with other living beings), the planet (the planet is a living ecosystem rather than inert matter), our understanding of time (which can be cyclical as well as linear), space (which can be understood not only in terms of the spaces of our gardens, but also in the relationships between this realm, the phases of the moon, and the cyclical phases of our bodies), and the process of change (change is needed not only outside ourselves but also within ourselves).

Because the need for this questioning of our personal/ political practices is so vital, I find myself with somewhat mixed emotions about the recent resurgence of interest in things "environmental," most visible in the growth of Green consumerism and the pageantry of Earth Summitry.[39] In the West, the radiation seepage from Chernobyl, the prospect of global warming, the discovery of an ozone hole, the ugliness of medical waste on ocean beaches, and the massive Exxon Valdez oil spill have lent a new sense of urgency to the "environmental crisis," contributing to the expansion of Green consumerism and the worldwide attention focused on the gathering of world leaders and environmental organizations at the Rio Summit of June 1992. Unfortunately, the profound ethical and political changes that would be necessitated by shifting our ecological worldview to see the earth as not primarily a resource for human projects are not represented in consuming ecologically friendly products, the wordings of environmental declarations signed by the leaders of nation states, or public opinion polls tapping greater support for environmental regulation. Indeed, environmental "management" is a rather old story, continuing the narrative of humans as being separate from nature with dominion over the Earth. The more efficient management of populations and resources has little to do with an engaged citizenry tending to their bioregions and the planet.

My concern with the form this new interest in the environment is taking is intensified when I am reminded of what population control has meant for the lives of women, especially in nations that have been designated as "overpopulated." Today, in the midst of a world where the peoples of the industrialized nations are gagging in the wastes of their consumption, the invocation of the population problem is particularly troublesome. The most recent "advances" in family planning techniques, from injectable contraceptives and vaccines against pregnancy to a range of hormonal implants, often banned in Western nations as unsafe, reduce women of the South to mindless objects and continue to imperialistically exploit native cultures "for their own good." That poor and often illiterate women are typically paid sums equal to the monthly wage of an agricultural worker when they become "acceptors of" either long-term contraceptives or sterilization (perhaps in an unsterile sterilization "camp") reveals that these women's contraceptive decisions have little to do with newfound freedom and are in fact the product of coerced choice.[40] The perverse logic of this model is especially visible when we see that most recently "new reproductive technologies" are being sold as a "boost" to India's sterilization program and as a valuable aid in producing, according to the patriarchal preference, boys.[41]

Ironically, the contemporary technical mastery of biological fertility, which the dominant culture promotes as a blessing and relief from the unwieldy sorrow and turmoil of the uncertainties of life, is the final point of instrumental thinking and economic logic. For when fertility is taken over by the specialist, isolated from the cyclical processes of the "natural world," patented and commodified, the cultural tissues that sustain life's vibrancy and joy are mutilated and destroyed. As Hannah Arendt (though neither a feminist nor an ecologist) so wisely noted,

> The human artifice of the world separates human existence from all mere animal environment, but life itself is outside this artificial world, and through life man remains related to all other living organisms. For some time now, a great many scientific endeavors have been directed toward cutting the last tie through which even man belongs among the children

of nature. It is the same desire to escape from imprisonment to the earth that is manifest in the attempt to create life in the test tube, in the demonstrated desire to mix "frozen germ plasm from people of demonstrated ability under the microscope to produce superior human beings" and "to alter (their) size, shape and function"; and the wish to escape the human condition.[42]

Arendt was writing when today's "new reproductive technologies," which allow some women to rent their wombs and others to choose which fetus they will bear, were still only a distant dream. My plea for a new life-affirming, democratic politics suggests that we also need to rethink some of the other cherished hopes that our technological management of life promises, from sex without consequences and children without turmoil, to food without sweat.

CHAPTER

3

SEX
WITHOUT
CONSEQUENCES:
FROM SEXUAL
FREEDOM
TO THE
SEXUATED BODY

It is odd that simply because of its "sexual freedom" our time should be considered extraordinarily physical. In fact, our "sexual revolution" is mostly an industrial phenomenon, in which the body is used as an idea of pleasure or a pleasure machine with the aim of "freeing" natural pleasure from natural consequence. Like any other industrial enterprise, industrial sexuality seeks to conquer nature by exploiting it and ignoring the consequences . . . and by evading social responsibility.

WENDELL BERRY,
The Gift of Good Land

Our culture obliges us to abandon all attempt to control our fertility by using our polymorphous potential for pleasure, and to give that control up to external agencies on the ground that they are both more efficient and less harmful. The efficacy of traditional methods has never been studied because they were invariably assumed not to exist.

GERMAINE GREER,
Sex and Destiny

When childbearing is not a punishment, but self-chosen, and when raising children is not an economic-survival disaster, most of us enjoy being around children. . . . But women don't always want children, for a multitude of reasons best determined by women. . . . When women are in natural control of our own fertility, population is always kept in practical relation to the needs of the group and the abundance of the environment. That, after all, is what it's all about.

MONICA SJOO AND BARBARA MOR,
The Great Cosmic Mother

WANT TO TURN NOW TO A MORE EXPLICIT CONSIDER-
ation of some of the cultural and political consequences of
the sexuated body, that is, the body defined exclusively by
sex. In an age when communities across the nation are seeking to banish gays and lesbians, I surely do not want to
argue that the preservation of sexual freedom is unimpor-
tant. At the same time, I am wary of some of the strategies
that have been taken up in the name of sexual freedom. My
concern here is the discourse regarding human biological
fertility in the contemporary United States and the relationship of that discourse to larger concerns about the fertility
of women internationally and the fertility of the Earth.

Identifying the Puzzle

In the late twentieth century, issues of sexuality constitute
some of the most divisive issues in United States politics.
The majority of voters continue to vote on the basis of traditional pocketbook issues such as taxes and the state of the
economy. Nonetheless, the most passionate conflicts, the
ones where everyone has a definite opinion, are over such
matters as contraceptive services for teenagers and state
regulation of abortion and homosexuality.

In 1981, the legislation which authorizes the budget for the United States government came perilously close to being stalled because of lack of agreement on a relatively tiny federal program—Title X of the Public Health Service Act—the federal government's major program of direct support for family planning services. In 1982, when the Secretary of the Department of Health and Human Services proposed a new regulation for Title X that would require notification of the parents of "unemancipated minors" who had received prescription drugs or devices at Title X clinics, the department was besieged with more letters and comments than it had received about any other single regulation in the history of the agency.

When the debate about whether teenagers should have access to contraceptives without their parent's knowledge hit the front pages, the liberal and leftist press as well as most of my friends read this debate as yet another instance of the forces of sexual repression rising up against the forces of sexual freedom. There is no doubt that the Reagan Administration represented a resurgence of the right in terms of nationhood, militarism, and glorification of the private market. At the same time, I felt then and still feel, that an interpretation stressing the sexual freedom/sexual repression dialectic does not adequately capture the complexity of the debates surrounding sexuality. The dominant story of women's situation has been that women are enslaved when they have no means of regulating their fertility. Alternative anthropological and historical data suggest, however, a more complicated narrative.[1]

Certainly grass-roots women in the South have been insistently declaring for the last few decades that their issues are access to land and water, adequate housing and transportation, and appropriate health care—the basics of survival, rather than the management objectives of family planners. But what of the argument that there is a clear distinction in terms of values and worldviews between birth control or reproductive rights on the one hand, and family planning on the other, that pioneering scholars such as Linda Gordon, Rosalind Petchesky, Betsy Hartmann, and activist across the globe have struggled to maintain?[2] And, perhaps most unsettling of all, what about modern birth control itself?

From Voluntary Motherhood to Birth Control

We can gain a perspective on the current conflicts in the United States from a consideration of nineteenth century women's movements before the modern welfare state had developed and before the terms "birth control" and "family planning" even existed. In the post Civil War period the women's movement in the United States, like today, contained a number of diverse groupings—suffragists, educational reformers, temperance advocates, social purity advocates and free-love advocates. While their causes were diverse, they were all united around their understanding of birth control. They promoted "voluntary motherhood," a philosophical and educational stance which approved of women choosing to limit their families at the same time that they condemned contraceptive devices as unnatural.[3] Rather than trying to explain their prudishness, I want to argue that the historically problematic aspects of the voluntary motherhood movements stem less from their attitudes about sexuality and contraception and more from their attitude about personhood and nurturance. A regime of safe sex produced by the fear of AIDS may have settled in some places, but our twentieth century, post-Freudian conditioning is still pervasive. Thus we identify easily the dangers of repression and the desirability of instant, unconstrained sex for both genders. Today, a stance advocating freedom for women that does not include modern forms of contraception seems nonsensical: unenlightened at best, and barbaric at worst. Before breathing a sigh of relief at how far we have come though, I want to look more closely at some of these nineteenth century reformers' arguments.

The attitudes toward sexuality held by the proponents of voluntary motherhood were not uniform. They varied from condemnations of male sexual abuse—both excessive or insensitive demands and physical violence—to support for the legitimacy of female sexual desire and the beauty of emotional and physical reciprocity. The voluntary motherhood reformers who extolled sexual expression always linked such discussions to the importance and necessity of moderation. "Free-lovers," who differed from the more moderate groups in their public opposition to a legal control of sexual behavior, nonetheless deplored what they termed "bondage to the passions."[4] Voluntary motherhood was to be achieved through women's independence from the sexual domination of her husband, and through male sexual restraint. The moral educator Lucinda Chandler, who was vice-president of the National Woman Suffrage Association and founded the Margaret Fuller Society to advocate both the education of women in the principles of government and the reform of the economic system, argued that

> The only true state of things is when the woman, as in all females in the animal kingdom, has control over her own person, independent of the desires of her husband. The imposition of the office of motherhood upon women in the 'old fashioned marriage,' regardless of her wish and fitness, has directly laid the foundation of the present instability and inharmony in marriage relations.[5]

For Chandler, self-ownership for women meant that women, not men, would decide when, where, and how sexual acts would be performed: "Women would no longer yield to unwarrantable intrusions upon her personal sanctity or be treated simply as an instrument for multiplying the species."[6] In short, voluntary motherhood rested not on the mastery of technique but on transforming the power relations between men and women.

The attempts of these reformers to bring honor and dignity to motherhood were intimately linked to their ideas about the well-being of children. For middle-class women in the burgeoning industrial economy of nineteenth century American, motherhood was emerging as a distinct and separate vocation in its own right. Initiating what was to be an important cultural shift, these reformers called attention to the value and significance of nurturing children and the attention and care that children needed if they were to flourish and grow. Nonetheless, immersed in nineteenth century conceptions of the natural, these reformers believed that the capacity for nurturance was strictly feminine. Their programs for change entailed no understanding that men were capable of nurturing.

The focus on nurturance was not unique to the reformers of the post Civil War period. It also shaped the ideology and practice of the women reformers of the Progressive Era who, in laboring for reforms intended to alleviate the poverty and dislocations of rapid industrialization, paved the way for the development of the American welfare state. Indeed, the argument that this generation of reformers made for suffrage centered on women's special strengths as nurturers and caretakers. Like their earlier sisters, these reformers also neglected the potential nurturing abilities of men. But they did make these qualities of caring central to their political program in their public espousal of the cause of female suffrage. Suffrage would be the mechanism through which women's talents and sensibilities could be extended to the public sphere.[7]

The question of what happened—or what failed to happen—in 1920 after women gained suffrage has been a source of controversy almost from the day the vote was achieved. Much of this debate is conducted with an eye to arguing that if reformers had chosen another strategy the promise of women's freedom might have already been realized. My concern in this book is not to discover the strategic mistakes of the 1920s, but rather to look at the transformations in the organization of knowledge that came to shape public policy. An understanding of how medical and therapeutic rationality took root during the 1920s can give us some insights into the available choices regarding women's economic well-being, health, and fertility regulation today.

The coalition of women reformers who achieved the suffrage victory, not surprisingly, used their new political clout to lobby immediately for a health care program for women and children. In 1921 Congress enacted, over the American Medical Association's heated protests, the Sheppard-Towner Maternity and Infancy Protection Act, the first federally funded social welfare program in the United States.[8] Its mandate was to reduce infant and maternal mortality through public health clinics, visiting nurses, consultation centers, childcare conferences, and literature distribution. Mothers were to be instructed in personal hygiene and methods of keeping their children healthy. As the historian Sheila Rothman writes, "Advances in health care were to come not from the construction of hospitals, medical research, or the training of medical specialists—or even from new cures for disease. Rather, educated women were to instill in other women a broad knowledge of the rules of bodily hygiene and in this way prevent the onset of disease."[9]

The cultural and economic context was changing, however, as the ideas of the European psychologists Sigmund Freud and Havelock Ellis were introduced to the United States. Madison Avenue saw early on that Freud's theories had a therapeutic use in helping the public overcome its guilt about ostentatious consumption. During the teens and twenties the development of American advertising produced a cultural industry which increasingly relied on what the historian Mary Ryan has termed the "sexy saleslady" to stimulate consumer desire for new goods.[10] As middle and upper class Americans generally took to various forms of psychoanalytic treatment, freedom and liberation came to be associated with the pleasure of sex. Repression, especially during what Freud called the "genital" phase of ego development, would lead inexorably to some combination of guilt, frigidity, and hysteria. In these shifting discourses of the body's pleasures and the family as a unit of consumption, Rothman notes that the appropriate realm for women shifted from the nursery to the bedroom.[11]

In 1915 Margaret Sanger, who was heavily influenced by Ellis's ideas about sexuality and the necessity of controlling the fertility of the poor, coined the term "birth control" and began to argue that contraception was "the key to the temple of liberty."[12] To Sanger, who argued against Sheppard-Towner, birth control could accomplish in one grand sweep all the different health, labor, and educational goals that the Progressive agenda sought to achieve through piecemeal reform. For Sanger, reduction in family size meant the end of poverty.

Some evidence suggests that Margaret Sanger's original concern was to provide women with basic information about hygiene and anatomy in clinics where nurses like herself would advise other women about these matters. In any case her program for women became transformed as she aligned herself with physicians and eugenicists. In 1918 a New York State Court ruled that only licensed physicians could provide contraception for the purpose of curing or preventing disease. Sanger moved from arguing for the free and unrestricted distribution of contraception to actively promoting the distribution of contraception through private physicians. Sexual practices became part of the doctor's domain, as birth controllers told women "ask your physician."[13]

As the medical profession consolidated its power during the 1920s, infant and maternity care became medicalized under the control of physicians just as contraception had.

Physicians argued that the possibility of abnormality in pregnancy was so great that it required intensive medical supervision. The role of public health nurses became sharply circumscribed as private physicians became increasingly interested in preventive health examinations. At Congressional hearings in 1929 which overturned Sheppard-Towner, physicians testified about pathologies of pregnancy and the potential ability of medical oversight and research to eliminate them. At the same time, the cultural and political shifts of the decade had taken their toll, undermining the once coherent political women's lobby that might have prevented the defeat of Sheppard-Towner.[14] The pervasive red-baiting of the period, signaled initially by the Palmer Raids of 1919, had a deleterious effect on the women's movement and social movements more generally. And these cultural shifts which undermined the women's lobby joined with the growth of psychoanalysis and the sexual objectification of women in advertising to produce the emergence of what I have termed the "sexuated" body.

The Institutionalization of Family Planning

Eugenicists had always been concerned about differential fertility rates between the "fit" and the "unfit." In the 1920s, as social workers, prison wardens, psychiatrists in prisons and mental asylums, and administrators of institutions for the alcoholics and the feebleminded provided expert testimony to state legislative bodies on the hereditary nature of social deviancy, eugenics was transformed from a creed into public policy. The British scientist Francis Galton, cousin to Charles Darwin, had first proposed in an 1865 article, "Hereditary Talent and Character," that human society could be improved by better breeding.[15] By the end of the 1920s thirty-two states had enacted sterilization laws which permitted compulsory sterilization of the unfit. As Ruth Hubbard and Elijah Wald note, "While the eugenicists diagnosed individuals with 'hereditary defects' in virtually all ethnic groups, they found that certain groups had a much higher proportion of 'defectives' than others. For this reason, eugenics was an explicit factor in the Immigration Restriction Act of 1924." The act served to decrease immigration to the United States from southern and eastern Europe in favor of persons with British and northern European descent.[16]

In the late 1930s, as many became deeply concerned about the western nations' falling rate of fertility, the term "family planning" emerged as a way of encouraging reproduction among the fit. As Margaret Sanger put it in 1939: "The eugenicists wanted to shift emphasis from less children for the poor to more children for the rich. We went back of that and sought first to stop the multiplication of the unfit. This appeared the most important and greatest step toward race betterment."[17] The need for family planning was increasingly emphasized within the larger historical goal of overall social planning. Linda Gordon reports in her *Woman's Body, Woman's Right* that a Birth Control Federation of America poster during this period reads "Modern Life is Based on Control and Science. We control the speed of our automobile. We control machines. We endeavor to control disease and death. Let us control the size of our family to insure health and happiness."[18]

Gordon and other scholars such as Rosalind Petchesky have seen this change in reproductive discourse as problematic primarily because of the shift to the family unit and the way in which family planning professionals and sex therapists focused on "marital fulfillment" and "family stability."[19] The issue of male power within the family that had been raised so forcefully by nineteenth century voluntary motherhood reformers was effectively ignored. But what is equally interesting here is the way in which sex was defined. Pleasure was constituted by heterosexual intercourse only, and sexual pleasure as an end unto itself was secured by modern forms of contraception which experts claimed afforded greater control and predictability. The patriarchal structure of the family did contain the sexually autonomous woman, but she was also contained by the sexual discourses within which this idea of sexual autonomy was constructed. This urban woman, who was more fully sexuated and industrialized than the nineteenth century voluntary mother, may have had access to a narrowed range of human pleasures, including sexual pleasure. The new discourse of family stability in the 1940s did nothing to fracture the logic of control and the mechanistic, reductionist worldview in which sexuality had become embedded.

As a public program, family planning continued to focus on controlling the births of poor women. Public spending for family planning was justified as reducing welfare expenses as well as the medical costs of maternity and newborn care, just as in the 1960s, when minimizing racial inequities became a focus of public concern, family planning would also be justified as helping to reduce differences in maternal and infant mortality rates between the races. As laboratory research produced ever newer technologies, the goal of family planners became one of ensuring that everyone had access to the most technologically advanced and effective contraception. Professional family planning counselors became necessary in order to assist people in "upgrading their practices." Survey data indicating that the white fertility rate had increased 50 percent over the 1930s, whereas the nonwhite fertility rate had increased 70 percent, intensified the call for maximizing access to the newest technologies.[20]

In the 1960s a national consensus on the need for family planning began to emerge with the new fear of a "population explosion." In 1961 the first Roman Catholic President, John F. Kennedy, delivered a foreign aid message to Congress declaring that population growth was threatening to outpace economic growth. In 1962, Deputy Assistant Secretary of State Richard N. Gardner, in an address to the United Nations General Assembly, offered American population assistance to nations that requested it. In 1965 President Lyndon B. Johnson announced that the Agency for International Development would "seek new ways to use our knowledge to help deal with the explosion in world population and the growing scarcity in world resources," and fourteen local Planned Parenthood chapters initiated family planning projects with War on Poverty funds. In his 1966 State of the Union message, Johnson included a commitment to funding for birth control programs at home and abroad, stating, "let us act on the fact that less than five dollars invested in population control is worth a hundred dollars invested in economic growth," and Congress amended the Foreign Assistance Act and the Food for Peace Act to "assist voluntary family planning programs in countries requesting such help." Foreign aid thus became contingent on host nations instituting family planning programs.

In 1967 the Economic Opportunity Act was amended to designate family planning as a "special emphasis project," and the Social Security Act was amended to *require* that states spend at least 6 percent of their maternal and child health funds on family planning services and that all AFDC recipients be offered family planning services. In 1969 President Richard Nixon sent a message to Congress requesting that "we establish as a national goal the provision of adequate family planning services to all those who want them but cannot afford them," and in 1970, with no testimony from the intended beneficiaries of the program and relatively little debate, the Congress passed the Family Planning Services and Population Research Act (Title X of the Public Health Service Act). A national family planning program was thus instituted at a time when the sharpest decline of fertility rates in American history had occurred over the previous thirteen years.

The constellation of forces that produced this consensus and its flurry of domestic and foreign policy activity cannot be completely untangled here. The United States' position in the changing world economy, with a concomitant increased dependence upon the labor, agricultural products, and natural resources of former colonial nations and an increased need to export and invest capital in these nations, created greater interest in influencing the growth rates there. Concurrently the migration of blacks in the Unites States from the agricultural South to the industrial centers of the urban North created anxiety concerning the availability of employment, housing, and other urban amenities. These shifts in demographics and the global economy undoubtedly contributed to an intensified focus on statecraft as the art of managing scarce resources. Some "critical" political economy explanations point to the role of corporate magnates in funding or staffing population research and advocacy projects that molded public consciousness in the post-World War II period, suggesting, either overtly or by implication, a capitalist scheme to hoard resources from the world's dispossessed peoples.[21]

The questions regarding equity, justice, and democratic participation that are raised by these shifts in American policy are crucially important. In particular, we must continue to examine the uneasy relationship between birth control advocacy and racist population control policies. At the same time it is important to note that during the mid 1960s the impetus for domestic family planning differed from the eugenics emphasis behind family planning prior to World War II. The Nazi atrocities during the war discredited eugenics for a new generation of planners. In the midst of the social turmoil that generated the Great Society, they were taken with the idea of using social engineering to eliminate poverty. For example, in 1966 during the height of the civil rights movement, a Department of Health Education and Welfare policy statement argued, "Family planning in the United States is an individual, health and social concern rather than a response to population pressures." The effects of this form of health advocacy supports population control efforts just as the pre-World War II reformers did, but the motivations of the different advocates should not be seen as unified. These differing motivations are of special relevance to the debate over adolescent pregnancy which was to emerge in the second half of the 1970s.

In comparison with domestic family planning, population control was a more explicit part of international family planning policy as it developed in the late 1960s. Paul Ehrlich's 1968 *The Population Bomb* played on people's fears of the chaos represented by the "teeming millions" of the South. Dr. R. T. Ravenholt, director of the newly created U.S. Office of Population, warned that revolutions endangering U.S. commercial interests would ensue if the population explosion remained unchecked. Yet even in the international arena, where U.S. aid programs were supplemented by newly created multilateral population agencies, population policy was not solely dedicated to impeding and containing foreign populations. Among professional family planners in the field, whose vision was fixed on poverty and pregnancy, emulating Sanger, family planning, including abortion (unlike Sanger), was viewed as the primary mechanism for alleviating misery and optimizing the well-being of the population.

Whether the goal was containment or optimization of well-being, women's bodies became the targets of the new cafeteria of contraceptive "choices" produced by a pharmaceutical industry that was always looking for new markets. In order to create a disciplined market that would find Western contraception desirable, family planning professionals utilized enticing media images that were most always supplemented by monetary and non monetary incentives. Women of the South were told "contraceptives are a woman's right." And if in a particular district an insufficient number of women became "acceptors," zealous recruiters, whose own survival within bureaucratic delivery systems depended on achieving their target goal, did not stop at tricking or compelling women to accept.[22]

Yet the family planning establishment's efforts to promulgate the dream of sex without consequences to the peoples of the South were a massive failure. To be sure, the promise of material goods and an improved standard of living, permitting ever larger numbers of people to imagine that the dream of food without sweat was in reach, has made "population control" a dominant ideal. But blindness to cultural diversity and the webs of relationships that sustain life often confound and obstruct even the best managed plans. As American family planning policies progressed, planners became aware that something was wrong with the family planning projects U.S. foundations had been encouraging in the developing world since the 1950s. The inundation of medical devices was not working, and supply was outstripping demand. At the World Population Conference in Bucharest in 1974, donors were heatedly criticized by the delegate from poorer nations: "they had done everything wrong: they had failed to integrate the people in their schemes, they had flouted ancient custom, they had ignored other basic needs such as infant nutrition and parasite control."[23]

The voluntary nature of participation in family planning programs became suspect during India's sterilization campaigns under Indira Gandhi's state of emergency in 1975; some family planners achieved their sterilization quotas by denying subsidies for irrigated water to villages that did not produce enough volunteers, while others threatened the unsterilized with fines and imprisonment. As criticisms of the Club of Rome's computer forecasts of impending world doom appeared, fear of the impending population explosion began to wane in the public mind. As it did so, and the growing mass movement against the 1973 Roe v. Wade

Supreme Court abortion decision returned public attention to the domestic scene, the stage was set for the next crisis—"teenage pregnancy."

The Adolescent as Client
and the Challenge to Family Planning

In 1976, after three years of declining budgets for Title X, The Alan Guttmacher Institute, the semi-independent research arm of the Planned Parenthood Federation (the organizational descendant of Margaret Sanger's work and the major group that had lobbied for federally supported health clinics with separate family planning services) issued a report entitled, *11 Million Teenagers: What Can Be Done About the Epidemic of Adolescent Pregnancies in the United States.* The report, with its reference to an epidemic conveying the sense of pregnancy as a rapidly contagious disease needing medical treatment, was widely circulated in the nation's media. The "disease" was one million adolescent pregnancies. The designated treatment group was not the pregnant adolescents themselves but rather the estimated 11 million sexually active teenagers between the ages of 15 and 19—7 million males and 4 million females.

In fact, contrary to the Guttmacher institute's suggestion, the birth rate among teenagers had actually declined substantially from its peak in the 1950s.[24] What had changed was the marital status of teenage mothers. Over the course of the seventies an increasing proportion of teenage births were occurring to unwed mothers (20.8 percent in 1965 compared to 38.2 percent in 1975). But perhaps equally significant from the standpoint of generating public concern were the reports that the rate of increase of unwed mothers was higher among white teenagers than among blacks. Unmarried teenage mothers were no longer perceived as an exclusively minority phenomenon. The main thrust of the

Guttmacher report was the need for more extensive family planning services—defined as access to sex education, birth control, and abortion, as well as the need for more federally supported research that would find the method of contraception that would work for teenagers.

The "crisis" of adolescent pregnancy was well publicized when Jimmy Carter came to office in 1977. In response, the Carter Administration focused on a "life-support" model rather than the family planning community's traditional prevention model. In broad terms this meant the prevention of unhealthy births and repeat pregnancies rather than pregnancy prevention per se. With its more holistic approach, the Carter Administration legitimized the idea that adolescents needed integrated and comprehensive services that were not exclusively medical. Nonetheless this shift was not framed as a direct challenge to the single service contraceptive approach to family planning that was the mainstay of the Title X program. That challenge would require a more significant political realignment than that of the Carter Administration.[25]

When Ronald Reagan came to office in 1981 he proposed to consolidate Title X into a health bloc grant to the states. Title X had been a particular object of concern for many of the constituencies that had contributed to Reagan's election. For some, Title X had come to signify the moral chaos and abuse of professional power that resulted from federal regulation of sexual matters. Although very few Title X clinics actually provided abortions, the association of Title X with abortion guaranteed the enmity of the New Right. Even more salient for this constituency was their belief that Title X allowed professional experts to provide teenagers and children with knowledge about sex that undermined the values and authority of parents. Though Title X had been passed as a family planning program for poor and low-income adult women, with the generation of ever increasing data on the sexual habits of ever more specific population groupings, media images that promoted the pleasure of sex and consumption, and the civil rights and sexual movements of the 1970s, unmarried teenage girls quickly became a significant population group for the program, both as actual clients and objects of outreach programs. Although most local sex education programs bore little direct relationship to Title X funds, this technical truth was of little relevance to critics who saw sex education health programs as the crucial vehicle by which the state subverted familial values.

Sentiments against Title X were strong. One group within the "pro-family" constituency argued that the government should get out of the family planning business. Another, led by Republican Senator Jeremiah Denton of Alabama, argued that the authority of the federal government should advocate a new approach to prevention—the prevention of sexual activity itself rather than simply the prevention of teenage pregnancy. Furthermore, services should be provided in a "family context." His proposal, which directly challenged the tenets of the established family planning community, quickly became popularized by the press as the "chastity act." The original draft of Denton's Adolescent Family Life bill called for the promotion of teenage "chastity" to curb adolescent "promiscuity," though the final bill called for the "promotion of self-discipline and other prudent approaches to the problem of adolescent sexual relations, including adolescent pregnancy."

The coalition of groups that supported the passage of the Adolescent Family Life Act was considerably more diverse than one might have expected. It included groups that had been intimately involved in the antiabortion, pro-life movement who insisted that the AFL bill would prohibit service providers from providing any information about abortion unless both a client and her parents requested it. But the coalition also included groups like the March of Dimes, the National Coalition of Hispanic Mental Health and Human

Service Organization and the Urban League. The Urban League supported the legislation because the legislations' care component, modeled after the 1978 Carter Adolescent Pregnancy Prevention Act, provided vitally needed social and medical services. High rates of adolescent pregnancy among blacks, in combination with the declining rates of pregnancy among older black women, rural to metropolitan migration, and the movement of middle-class blacks out of urban ghettoes, had created a situation in which an increasing proportion of black babies came into the world outside the supportive neighborhood and extended kin networks that had historically sustained the black community. Moreover, the AFL bill's focus on abstinence and male responsibility met with receptivity among leaders in minority communities. With the shifting structure of the economy, and with the larger culture's sanctioning of the sexuated body, many minority adolescents began to find a large part of their meaningful self-definition in the number of children they bore.

The parental involvement amendment was a Congressional compromise struck in response to efforts to require parental consent. It was left to Health and Human Services to implement the meaning of "encouraging involvement." In February of 1982 the department proposed regulations requiring that the parents or guardian of unemancipated minors age seventeen or under be notified if prescription drugs or devices had been provided to such minors. The regulation quickly became known as "the squeal rule" through the national media and, as I mentioned earlier, the department was besieged with an unprecedented number of letters and petitions.

The anxieties and hopes this proposed regulation generated intrigued and troubled me. Curious about the character of the expressed sentiments, I decided to venture into an HEW storage room to peruse the responses the department actually received.[26] Not surprisingly, all but a handful of the letters from physicians, therapists, and social workers opposed the regulation. Comments in support of the regulation came largely from nonprofessionals and active church members. Most letters on both sides came from women, but men were more likely to oppose the mandated parental involvement. Petitions in opposition almost always included both males and females, whereas petitions among the supporters (petitions and handwritten letters were also more common on this side) were almost always completely female. If men appeared at all, they appeared as spouses.

Examining the voices that were represented in these letters, it became increasingly clear that the sexual freedom/sexual repression dialectic simply fails to capture the complicated layers of the debate around adolescent sexuality in this country. For example, those who opposed parental notification frequently emphasized the costs of welfare systems. They argued that if more barriers were placed between potential contracepting clients and services, those clients would become welfare clients. To the extent that the question of cost was raised by the supporters of parental involvement, it was only because parents would be responsible for the medical costs of potential complications of contraception and therefore should be consulted about their children's contraceptive decisions. The professional opponents often mentioned the difficulties adolescents have in talking with parents, whereas the citizen supporters were more likely to mention the rights and responsibilities.

These letters led me toward a different vantage point on this debate. Perhaps parents who support parental notification regulations are not all merely insisting on asserting familial authority and prudish ideas regarding sexuality. They may also be seen as protesting the hierarchies of truth and value that have been created by professional experts. I cannot help but wonder whether the cause of freedom and democratic politics is always advanced by unequivocally supporting the scientific truths of professionals seeking to maintain their position against the truths of ordinary parents who have been deemed parochial and unenlightened.

In any case, the issue today is not simply how to talk about sex, the challenge that is being raised by the advocates of the new prevention approach, but rather how to, in Foucault's terms, "end the monarchy of sex." His comments regarding children are especially interesting here and could be seen as being supportive of the more complicated notions of pleasure, truth, and attachment that are contained within ecofeminist discourse.

> Look at what is happening as far as children are concerned. Some say: children's life is their sex life. From the bottle to puberty, that's all it is. Well, are you sure that this type of discourse is actually liberating? Are you sure that it doesn't lock children into a sort of sexual insularity? And what after all if they just couldn't care less? If the liberty of not being an adult consisted exactly in not being enslaved to the law of sexuality . . . would it be so boring after all? If it were possible to have polymorphic relationships with things, people and bodies, wouldn't that be childhood? To reassure themselves, adults call this polymorphic perversity, coloring it thus with the monotonous monochrome of their own sexuality.[27]

Beyond Family Planning

The contemporary conflicts around family planning cannot be accounted for by traditional left/right political dichotomies. In particular, women's voices are on both sides of the conflict. The languages of control and hierarchy permeate both the arguments of those who argue for freedom and choice and those who talk of family and authority. Family planning as it is deployed across the globe produces ever more complicated mechanisms for reconstructing women's bodily cycles and preparing bodies for entry into the world of consumer pleasures.

What is particularly troublesome from a feminist perspective is, again, how the feminist goal of controlling our bodies, embedded as it is in the language of rights and choice, is inscribed within the discourse about family planning.[28] As I have already argued, in the context of the particular confluence of science, sex, and power that mark contemporary capitalist societies, the language of controlling the body tends to strengthen those cultural patterns which narrow our understandings of pleasure and our bodies to sex. One of the more serious political consequences of this narrowing of identity is the undermining of the cultural grounding for egalitarian relations, and democratic politics more generally, making it difficult, if not impossible, to cultivate awareness of the manifold nature of the human capacity for pleasure, our common ties with each other, and the multitude of living creatures with whom we share the earth.

I have focused here on traditional family planning. The need for alternatives that can resist the normalizing powers of medicine, science, and education becomes even more compelling when we consider the dilemmas raised by "new family planning"—the early detection of physical defects through prenatal screening, extrahuman fertilization techniques like in vitro fertilization and embryo transfer; and the possibilities of genetic engineering that loom on the horizon. The enticements of new reproductive technologies may hold some promise of eliminating sorrows, but they also hold the possibility of creating new sorrows for generations yet unborn. We must develop ethical guidelines grounded in the connective webs that sustain life without at the same time reinforcing traditional gender hierarchy and exploitation.

In creating new, or renewed understandings of bodies and pleasure we need to focus less on acts of coitus and more on the nature of human expression and our species' manifold sensuous connections with the world. With respect to heterosexual pleasures, sexual practices infused with some sense of lunar fertility awareness (most especially practices that resist the grip of the outside expert) hearken back to the wisdom of the voluntary motherhood reformers, as they create the potential for a more woman-centered, participatory, and ecologically mindful world.

Today fertility awareness has arisen primarily in the context of natural family planning or natural birth control, both in grass-roots religious communities and the holistic health movement. As a way of creating procreative choice, practices of birth prevention such as awareness of mucous secretions or basal body temperature have much to recommend them. As a way of fostering self-knowledge, reading bodily signs that change with the phases of the menstrual cycle helps to reduce dependence on medical expertise and no-think technologies. Women, whatever their age, practicing these forms of body awareness learn to read their particular fertility cycle and become attuned to changes in their body. These practices can thus facilitate early detection of many illnesses and hold the potential of producing healthier women who have less need of the most complicated medical and pharmaceutical technologies. The cancers, immune system disorders, and assorted reproductive disorders of DES daughters and sons whose mothers took this drug to ward off miscarriage is only one of the painful reminders that the prevailing conception of health and medical effectiveness in our country is a short-term one which ignores the issue of sustainability across generations.[29] Furthermore, because fertility awareness practices as a method of contraception can only be effective when male partners are conscious of the cycles of women's bodies, they may also hold the potential of more egalitarian gender relations.[30]

But fertility awareness as a practice of daily life is perhaps most promising as a way to cultivate recognition of the complex connections between the fertility of our bodies and the fertility of the Earth. For example, recent evidence suggests that both female and male infertility have important environmental components. The same is true for spontaneous abortions, ectopic pregnancies, the birth of handicapped newborns, contaminated breast milk, and breast and prostatic cancer.[31] And around the world, famine and hunger often result in large part from industrialized agricultural production which fails to nurture and care for the soil.[32] Such problems, and the heroic and invasive techniques typically offered as solutions, are by-products of our modern ideology of control, which has little respect or awe for the lunar cycles of the earth.[33]

It is important to note here that modern forms of contraception beginning with the barrier methods totally divorce birth prevention from the facilitation of conception. This fracturing of fertility practices is reflected in the dominant discourse which tends to frame the question of choice as the choice not to procreate. In contrast, fertility awareness practices can be used for both birth prevention and the facilitation of conception, using modern biology to create a more holistic approach to fertility, similar to the practices of nonmodern societies. Angus MacLaren, in *Reproductive Rituals,* for example, demonstrates that in early modern England the same practices used to promote fertility were also used to restrict fertility. Midwives rather than male doctors were the primary transmitters of this knowledge.[34]

Whereas population control and family planning focus on individuals, contributing to social isolation, excessive professionalism, and the standardization of norms of bodily perfection, ecological discourses of the body and planet infused with fertility awareness could expand our understandings of conviviality, responsibility and the sacredness of life, allowing us to resist the promised freedoms of population control planners and high-tech agricultural planners. We must move beyond the mechanistic view of nature that has sought to dominate and exploit the natural world since the dawn of the modern era.

Abortion and the Cycles of Life

Today, many who advocate fertility awareness—most especially those who see this awareness as primarily a contraceptive technique and seek to institutionalize it within international family planning programs—would also have the state ban abortion. There are even some within this loose constellation, both women and men who think of themselves as feminists, who argue that because feminism is about nonviolence, feminism and moral or legal support of abortion are incompatible. The connection between feminism and nonviolence is integral to ecofeminist politics, but if nonviolence is to be brought into discussions of the state and the regulation of abortion, as I think it should, we must also attend to the violence that is entailed in the bureaucratic prescriptions that are the contemporary state.

While I do not accept the contention that abortion necessarily constitutes violence, my own experiences of pregnancy and birth have also made me aware that there can be an underside to the legal sanctioning of abortion. I have often wondered about how radically different my own life might have been if I had not found myself unexpectedly pregnant as I finished my applications for graduate school in the days before Roe v. Wade. My sense is that given my particular life goals, I might well have never experienced the wonder of life that parenting can bring. I am also aware that the extra energy I derived from being both student and mother seemed to come so "naturally" because I had a partner who was especially intrigued by the opportunities of parenting. I was extremely lucky. Yet because of what I did learn about myself and the needs of children, I still find myself a bit troubled when I hear of highly educated women on the way to better careers and opportunities who "know" that an unplanned pregnancy will ruin their life. While these women are surely materially advantaged, I find myself wondering if such women are spiritually advantaged in comparison to the women they often seek to help and advise. At the same time I have absolutely no interest in either the state banning or regulating abortion. I concur with Catharine MacKinnon that to recognize the fetus as a form of life does not logically necessitate a political stance against the legality of abortion.[35]

MacKinnon's argument for why women must have the legal right to decide about abortion is grounded in a decidedly different worldview than the more conventional pro-choice stance that argues against state interference on the grounds of privacy and individual rights. Indeed, for MacKinnon, the Roe v. Wade decision that legalized abortion by finding that criminal statutes violated a legal right of privacy embodied in law what she terms a "male point of view." She argues that in the context of sexual intercourse that is not "coequally determined," privacy doctrine merely "keeps some men out of the bedrooms of other men."[36] This insistence on bringing to the fore the male coercion that may have produced a pregnancy is important and helps to differentiate a feminist argument for the availability of abortion from arguments that focus on the right of physicians not to have their professional judgment second-guessed by the state.

At the same time this foregrounding of men's domination and control of women's sexuality does not necessarily lead to a pro-choice political stance. Feminists for Life, for example, share with MacKinnon a stance toward abortion that emphasizes male coercion, characterizing "abortion as something forced on many women by a male-dominated society." For the philosopher and writer Celia Wolfe-Devine, who argues against abortion from what she terms an ecofeminist perspective, "The masculine tendency is to emphasize control, domination and technological manipulation of nature, rather than living in harmony with it. And this is the root of our ecological crisis. . . . abortion clearly violates the rhythms and cycles of nature."[37] Thus we see that premises such as MacKinnon's that highlight the abusiveness of men can be made to move in different directions. On the one hand, such premises may support a pro-choice stance which finds the logic of Roe v. Wade insufficiently sensitive to male supremacy. On the other hand, some religious ecofeminists, who also understand the issue of abortion in the context of patriarchy, would choose to use the state to protect women from what they see as the inherent abusiveness of abortion.

My own view of the complicated issues of abortion is that while an ecofeminist perspective affirms the intricate web of life, it also cautions that efforts to preserve life must necessarily accept that both birth and death are integral to the cycles of nature. Thus, for example, many fertilized eggs are not successfully implanted. Why some live and some do not is part of the mystery of life. Thus for ecofeminists, to be "for life" is to honor the fact that renewal and growth is intimately related to periods that are fallow. In contrast, modern science, in its unceasing effort to exert greater control over the processes of life, refuses to accept the basic wisdom that humans are mortal, that death cannot be conquered. Indeed the vast institutional array of medical and biotechnological power in modern societies invite us to imagine otherwise. Thus we find that our earthly fate is consistently disguised by benign counselors and physicians whose mission it is to defer our acknowledgment of death and the finitude of human existence.

From an ecofeminist perspective, I hold no illusion of triumph over death and am sensitive to the operations of contemporary power. The preservation and harnessing of life as it is practiced by contemporary scientific experts often thwarts the spontaneity and unruliness that characterize human life. In my view the pro-choice position that typically argues abortion would not be necessary if better birth control were available, and the conventional pro-life position that argues abortion is never justified because all life must be preserved in all circumstances, are each merely variants of this curious modern notion that death and sorrow can be banished through better management and control. Thus these seemingly antithetical political stances share considerably more than one might imagine at first glance. Each, despite drawing different inferences regarding the implications of a logic of control, accepts the fundamental premise of this logic regarding the contingencies of human existence.

In contrast to this managerial approach to the uncertainties and flux of living, the ecofeminist approach to fertility that I am calling for does not ask for chance to be eliminated. Ecofeminists do not glorify risk; but their interest in minimizing risk is chastened by the knowledge that to too insistently order nonconformity and mystery is to squelch life itself. Accepting the basic feminist contention that women should have no less moral agency than men, ecofeminists insist that women be recognized as agents who are capable of making the life and death decisions that necessarily arise in an imperfect world. Ecofeminists cultivate the personal, spiritual, and social relations that enable women to welcome the gift of life, but individual women still must be the ones to decide whether to carry a particular pregnancy to term.[38]

This reliance on women's decision-making capabilities does not stem from any natural right women have to control their bodies that necessarily supersedes all connections a biological father has to a developing fetus; rather, women's agency with respect to abortion is grounded in the sober and pragmatic assessment that all other rules for governing the abortion decision enhance the power of an already intrusive and bureaucratic state. Notions of "mother-right" are appealing as alternatives to the historical abuses of patriarchal power, but they are ultimately inadequate for building a democratic politics that is respectful of the contingencies of life. Recognizing the importance of democratic politics to these most intimate decisions also helps us to be mindful of the places on the planet where abortion and the most technologically advanced forms of contraception may be freely available and uncontested, yet women are still not acknowledged as moral agents.

While both the criminalization and regulation of abortion by state authorities must always be resisted, it is equally important to remember that in the contemporary world, population politics, the manipulation of people as faceless numbers, is usually more appealing than democratic politics. Nation states that legalize abortion often do so for a variety of reasons that have little to do with the moral integrity of women. These reasons of state are often difficult to discern when elites readily pose abortion or technologically advanced contraception as the fertility control that is integral to women's freedom. In the contemporary world the language of controlling our bodies does not necessarily challenge masculinist power and can easily become a principle of regulation which sustains that power.

CHILDREN WITHOUT TURMOIL: FROM SEX WITHOUT REPRODUCTION TO REPRODUCTION WITHOUT SEX

For us women, for nature, and for the people of developing nations, this technology is a declaration of war. . . . The human- and nature-despising character of this technology reveals itself in the reduction of human and nonhuman living organisms to a few exploitable properties and functions. Once we fall into the double trap of the technology's power and our mere ability to make it happen, living organisms are going to be arbitrarily constructed, changed, and improved, without any regard for the far-reaching consequences of such activity for life on earth. Spontaneity, vivacity, nonconformity—in short, the multi-faceted character of all life, including human life—will thus become factors which disrupt the production process.

Resolution from 1985 conference,
"Women Against Genetic Engineering
and Reproductive Technologies" (Germany)

Our ecological consciousness which has awakened of late, has awakened because of the realization that ultimately it is we who are going to suffer if plundering of resources is not checked. Yet we have to evolve much more before we actually learn to coexist instead of blindly trying to control. What has happened and is happening to women's reproductive ability is something very similar.

CHAYANIKA, SWATIJI AND KAMAXI,
We and Our Fertility

It is not that life has been totally integrated into techniques that govern and administer it; it constantly escapes them. Outside the Western world, famine exists, on a greater scale than ever; and the biological risks confronting the species are perhaps greater and more serious, than before the birth of microbiology. . . . Modern man is an animal whose politics places his existence as a living being in question.

MICHEL FOUCAULT,
The History of Sexuality

WITH THE BIRTH OF LOUISE BROWN, THE WORLD'S first "test-tube baby," in Great Britain in July 1978, discussion of alternative forms of conception moved from the pages of science fiction and medical journals to the headlines of newspapers and news magazines across the globe.

The media have fastened on the human intrigue, legal puzzles, and medical heroics of producing babies without traditional coitus. For example a September 1991 *Time* cover story, "Making Babies" discusses the happiness of a forty-eight year old South African postmenopausal woman who was the first woman to give birth to her own grandchildren, serving as a surrogate for her daughter who had lost her uterus. The article also points out different legal dilemmas such as whether "embryos, frozen or thawed, have a legal right to life" but then argues that these ethical questions "pale before the newly revealed miracle of fertilization, an event so complex that researchers say the more they understand it, the more they wonder that it works as often as it does. . . . The beauty and power of IVF is that it allows doctors to take many key events in reproduction out of the body, where they are subject to the vagaries of human biology, and perform them in-vitro—'in glass.'"[1]

Of course the miracle of life is not newly revealed by the techniques of infertility researchers. What is new is the emphasis on improvement of the miracle. The article in *Time,* for instance, also discusses how the basic IVF procedure has been improved by two variants, GIFT, or gamete intrafallopian transfer, and ZIFT, zygote intrafallopian transfer. The "advantages" of these newer procedures is that the implantation rate is higher than that of traditional IVF. At a clinic using these newest procedures, a single cycle "can result in pregnancy 40% to 50% of the time." In contrast, "A healthy, fertile couple trying to conceive naturally in any given month will have about a 25% success rate."[2] The implied conclusion is that nature is much too sloppy and inefficient.

From an ecofeminist perspective, this emphasis on technological mastery is particularly disturbing. First, we need to take account of how the medical heroics of saving life, and now *producing* life, is necessitated by the ecological threats to well-being our very mode of living continually produces. Greater interventions to cure the diseases endemic to industrialism serve to obscure precisely those degrading, toxic practices that point toward ecocide. Indeed, one of the arguments of this chapter is that new reproductive technologies and genetic engineering, by ameliorating the raw edge of progress, are themselves fully implicated in the stability of industrial practices. Second, we also need to take account of how this system of medical heroics joins with the general impulse throughout our culture to control fertility and so improve our lives. The cumulative effects of such "improvements" can produce social and ecological consequences that threaten life itself.

Let me explore this second point first. Central to new reproductive technologies and, lately, embryonic technologies is the logic that since the eighteenth century has sought to take charge of life by bringing "life and its mechanisms into the realm of explicit calculations."[3] New realms of regulation and surveillance are constantly created. Foucault argues that over the course of the nineteenth century the medicalization of women's bodies "was carried out in the name of the responsibility they owed to the health of their children, the solidity of the family institution, and the safeguarding of society."[4] Today, women's birthing bodies are reconfigured in gynecologists' offices and hospital wards, every facet of procreation commodified and monitored in the name of health and choice. Doctors, genetic counselors, biomedical research scholars, and lab technicians divide bodies into ever smaller and more malleable parts. These experts have learned how to splice a living person into an endless variety of combinations which are then distributed in a market of human pieces across time and space that defy what had hitherto been accepted biological constraints.

In the late twentieth century, with the majority of women in the West already in the paid labor market, we see how these new medical techniques have redefined the "productivity" of women's bodies. An ever-growing pharmaceutical industry requires living material such as eggs, embryos, and fetal tissue for a variety of life-saving purposes, a situation which has led some critics to raise a number of morally sordid scenarios. The feminist theorist Jean Elshtain, for example, has raised the specter of a new form of pregnancy for hire in which fetal tissue will be harvested from aborted fetuses and implanted in the brains of Parkinsons patients in order to stem the course of this degenerative disease.[5] Other scenarios project women being induced into later abortions so as to produce the "best" tissue for a variety of life-saving purposes.[6] Such concerns are not unreasonable. Nonetheless, these dramatic scenarios can obscure an even more worrisome threat: the efforts of contemporary experts to help all women have their "own" healthy babies. The miracles of modern science and the rise of the surrogacy industry have made this apparently benign goal an issue fraught with complex difficulties, leading to problems which even Solomon could not answer.

Surrogacy, Fertility, and Ecological Degradation

In 1986, when Mary Beth Whitehead, a "surrogate moth-er," decided she did not want to turn over the baby she had contracted to produce for William and Elizabeth Stern, a dramatic custody battle ensued. Who were the "rightful" parents of Baby M? This question immediately transcended the purely legal domain, generating worldwide intrigue and the call for new policies that would enable society to come to grips with the realities of biomedical advance. In this new world of reproduction without sex, feminists vainly strug-gled to maintain the principle of a woman's right to control her body. But feminism's attachment to the logic of control —the effort to rein in the vagaries of life's fortunes through scientific or legal predictability—made it difficult to develop a coherent response to the Baby M case. In this instance the logic of control could be marshalled by either side.

On the side of opportunity, it was argued that women had fought long and hard to gain the right to enter into contracts. Some feminist lawyers welcomed the new tech-nologies, claiming that efforts to weaken a woman's right to rent her womb would reinforce the historic view of women as fickle and irrational. Moreover, the contemporary femi-nist movement had labored to uncouple motherhood and personhood, calling on men to actively participate in par-enting. To argue that Mary Beth Whitehead had an origi-nary and inviolable "maternal" tie with this baby would reinforce the worst patriarchal constructions of woman-hood: that our most important, indeed only, role is that of mother. Feminist opposition to the new reproductive options, in a period where women's right to abortion was being contested, would serve to weaken the legitimacy of women's reproductive freedom. For the lawyer Lori Andrews, surrogacy "was a natural outgrowth of the wom-en's movement."[7] In the past two decades women had begun to pursue educational and career possibilities previously reserved for men. In doing so, many had also postponed childbearing. As many discovered that the chance for a child had slipped by, they "needed to turn to a surrogate mother."[8] Within this framework it was the concerns of Elizabeth Stern that needed support.

There were also many who were drawn to the plight of the birth mother. Many feminists charged that surrogacy was a new variant of men's control over women. For Janice G. Raymond, "The act of men buying women for sex bears a striking resemblance to men buying women's reproductive services in surrogacy."[9] For many there was something deeply patriarchal and bourgeois about the contention that the well off and educated Sterns could provide this child a level of security that would not be available in the home of her lower-middle-class and single biological mother. Mary Beth Whitehead's consent to rent her womb could not be separated from the choices generally available to lower and working-class women. William Stern's desire to purchase a baby with his own genes had enabled him to exploit Mary Beth Whitehead in the time-honored tradition of men seeking certainty of their paternity. Others argued that the effort to put the bond between mother and child on the level of contract law denied the personhood of women, contributing to their dehumanization. Some further suggested that Elizabeth Stern's reputed inability to bear a child disguised her desire not to disrupt her well-established career as a doctor and medical school professor with a pregnancy.

In 1991 the U.S. Supreme Court determined in Automobile Workers v. Johnson Controls that the exclusion of fertile women from a battery manufacturing plant in Wisconsin constituted sex discrimination.[10] Though the issues in this case are ostensibly rather different from those of Baby M, the near universal feminist celebration of this decision serves to underscore the dilemmas contemporary feminism increasingly finds itself in. With this case, where twenty or thirty million women would have faced job discrimination because of the adoption of fetal protection policies in hazardous workplaces, feminists were not as openly divided as in the case of Baby M. Here the feminist legal community was united around the right of women workers at Johnson Controls to work in a toxic environment. Women had struggled to enter the field of well-paying, albeit hazardous, jobs and they would not allow biomedical understanding of procreation to form a new rationale for women's exclusion. The available evidence indicated that lead exposure could have a debilitating effect on the male reproductive system, but men were not similarly excluded; indeed one of the plaintiffs was a man who had been denied a request for a leave of absence for the purposes of lowering his lead level because he intended to become a father. In a political context where women's right to abortion was increasingly attacked through pitting fetuses against women, the Supreme Court decision was viewed as a victory for women. But as the historian Ruth Rosen noted, "The freedom to endanger one's life and potential offspring is a hollow victory. . . . I am delighted that women will not have to choose between sterilization and gainful employment. Winning was certainly better than losing. But this was no feminist victory. This is a dystopian nightmare."[11] The perversity of the Johnson verdict is made clearer when we realize that when women who have won the right to work in toxic workplaces do conceive they will likely be encouraged to abort defective fetuses that sonograms and genetic screening procedures may disclose.

The Baby M and Johnson Control cases, however dramatic, deflect attention from the far less controversial instances of helping infertile women have babies in their own bodies and of helping all mothers have "normal" babies. I believe it is within these relatively invisible processes of biomedical monitoring and surveillance such as now routine ultrasounds, blood screenings, and amniotic fluid testing, processes we so freely accept, that the greatest threats to human life lie. The vast mosaic of medical records collected from this monitoring across generations may only further the homogenization of identities, as the meaning of being human becomes the possession or lack of proliferating disease categories. Having a "healthy" baby will no longer be seen as a gift of good fortune, but as the result of correct screening and testing.

Many feminists were outraged by William Stern's efforts to obtain a baby with his own genes. Yet the enticements of technological life-enhancement are so compelling that many of those outraged by Stern also leveled comparable disgust at the restrictions which impede federal support of infertility research. The irony is that the commodification of life that so many found abhorrent in the case of Baby M is considerably more advanced, some might argue constitutive of the process, in the biomedical research industry that supports everyday infertility and genetic counseling.

A crueler irony is that the more we focus on the fertility problems of humans and ignore the ways in which we are poisoning the Earth, the more we move toward a world where the complete and total control of baby-making by medical experts is considered prudent and wise. The conception and birth of a healthy child on a thoroughly poisoned earth is likely to be so problematic that the choice of nonintervention will be totally lost. Technologically produced babies will become the order of the day.

The scenario I have painted is not a particularly appealing one to say the least. One might very well argue that it is beside the point, indeed meaningless, to speculate about what birth would be like when the Earth is fully poisoned, since it is highly unlikely that women or men would be alive if the Earth was no longer alive. (Considering that most evidence suggests that the Earth can live without us, while we cannot live without it, my hunch is that a poisoned Earth would live on without the "benefit" of one of its species.)

My reason for engaging in such seemingly silly speculations is to bring the issue of new reproductive technologies out of the narrow medical and legal contexts in which it is typically discussed and into an arena where it is possible to see the links between the fertility of women, the well-being of babies, and the well-being of the Earth. The push to regulate and monitor, which emerges in varying degrees from the interests of medical researchers, lawyers, doctors, genetic counselors, and the anxieties of client-consumers, typically assumes that the birth of healthy babies is a function of equitably distributed diagnostic medicine. The notion that the health of individual bodies is related to the health of the social body and the ecosystem that sustains us recedes far into the background as experts focus on the microcomponents of procreation and birthing.

Genes, Normalization, and the Language of Control

To date the routinization of procedures such as amniocentesis (in which a needle is inserted into a mother's abdomen to extract amniotic fluid for the purpose of detecting information about the chromosomal structure and sex of the fetus) and other prenatal and antenatal diagnostic technologies has evolved from largely voluntary practices. In a cultural context that presumes modern technological medicine can guarantee the birth of "perfect" babies, pregnant women and physicians both seek to reduce risks and uncertainties. On one side, mothers seek to reduce anxieties and fears that have been heightened by the increased number of tests for abnormalities. On the other, physicians seek to allay those fears and protect themselves against malpractice suits by advising women to take advantage of the best available tests. This biomedical environment has reshaped pregnancy, creating what the sociologist Barbara Katz Rothman has termed the "tentative pregnancy," in which many women do not allow themselves to experience the bodily murmurs indicating new life, disallowing any identification with their changing body until a medical expert has assured them that their fetus is "normal."[12] To date shifting standards of sound medical practice, rather than formal state guidelines, have been the primary shaping force in the routinization of pre-natal quality control mechanisms such as amniocentesis, ultrasound imagery, and alpha-feto protein testing (a simple blood test for detecting neural tube defects).

It is this context that makes recent genetic screening legislation in California, often a leader in policy innovation, particularly noteworthy. California chose to initiate a statewide alpha-feto protein screening program in 1986 when the President's Commission for the Study of Ethical Problems had recommended against the routine screening of all pregnant women.[13] To some observers California's rush to mass screening was pushed by the large number of existing genetic centers in California which would prosper as the client base grew. Whatever the shaping forces, and despite the fact that it is too early to assess the actual impact of this effort to directly wed state policy to the advances of seemingly benevolent prenatal technologies, the launching of the program highlights some of the complicated questions regarding individual choice, normalization, and societal responsibilities that are raised by the practice of prenatal screening technologies more generally.

One of the particularly interesting features of the California screening program is the way in which it builds on the "voluntariness" that characterizes the existing genetic counseling system to induce mass participation. Prenatal care providers in California are required to provide all their patients with a state-prepared brochure that discusses the screening program for anecephaly and spina bifida. Voluntary participation in the program is emphasized by bold type; if a woman does not want to have the test, she is asked to sign an informed refusal statement, which reads "I

REFUSE to have the AFP blood screening test done. I understand and accept the consequences of this decision." Thus, in addition to mandating informed consent, a fairly routine practice in genetic counseling systems, the program also provides for a version of what might be termed informed refusal.

Because the program is so new, how the courts and insurance companies will treat persons who are born with neural tube defects in instances where their mothers have refused the test remains to be seen. Will insurance companies, for example, argue that they are not liable for the expenses of treatment? It is worth noting the arguments of the State Commissioner of Genetic Services regarding the cost-saving features of the program, who commented that "if 90 percent of women found to be carrying severely malformed babies choose abortions, $13.3 million will be saved statewide in lifetime medical costs for every 100,000 women screened and $3.7 million will be saved for Medi-Cal."[14] Will such reasoning lead to the erosion of support services for persons with special needs and the devaluation of the lives of the living who have "wrong" chromosomal structures? Will courts permit children to sue their mothers for wrongful life, to sue for having been born? The availability of written evidence regarding the mother's refusal to take advantage of available medical procedures raises the specter of mothers being sued for "negligence." The results of this apparently beneficent technology for which democratic access has been made available may be ambiguous at best.

Yet, most women will probably enter the system. As Ruth Hubbard insightfully comments, "as long as childbearing is privatized as women's individual responsibility and as long as bearing a disabled child is viewed as a personal failure for which parents (and especially mothers) feel shame and guilt, pregnant women are virtually forced to hail medical "advances" that promise to lessen the social and financial burdens of bearing a disabled child."[15] What is neglected in

California's complex screening plan is the acknowledgement that ordinary low-tech prenatal care and nutrition care, typically the best prevention for birth defects, are not covered, nor, for that matter, are they particularly well covered by other state pregnancy programs. The expenditure of resources for a complicated screening program may actually divert needed resources from a system already strained to meet the prenatal needs of low-income women.

It is these larger cultural and political contexts that point to the moral paradoxes of high-tech approaches to pregnancy and birth that focus on inherited diseases. Helping individual women to avoid bearing children with disabilities can weaken a society's commitments and responsibilities to those living people who because of poverty or disabilities (whether acquired through inheritance or the accidents of living) require special support. Advocates for persons with disabilities question the medicalized view of disability as a tragedy and ask further what the much heralded ability to conquer disabilities through encouraging women not to bear babies with disabilities means for the value of the lives of persons with disabilities.[16] While proponents of screening argue that access to advanced technology is necessary to ensure either the right to bear healthy children or the right to be born healthy, critics argue that routine prenatal screening medicalizes every pregnancy and nourishes eugenic ideologies. In Germany, where the memory of Nazism is tenacious, feminist have been vociferously critical and organized in their response to the new reproductive technologies, focusing on their inscription in a new, subtler eugenics.

In the United States, and the West more generally (with the exception of Germany), the feminist response to the new reproductive technologies has been considerably more enthusiastic. The few critics such as Gena Corea and Renata Duelli Klein have tended to characterize the newest stage of reproductive technology as yet another stage in the age-old male supremacist war against women's reproductive powers. These activists and critics have raised important questions about the invasiveness of in-vitro fertilization and the desires of scientists to test their techniques simply because it was possible. They have been assiduous in ferreting out information on the risks and dangers of the surgeries and hormonal drugs the new infertility treatments necessitate. They point to the risks posed for women's long-term health and the health of any offspring. They also point to the physical and psychological trauma women experience in fertility clinics and the low actual birth rate, the disjuncture between promise and performance.[17] Their critiques underscore both the masculinist character of the new reproductive technologies and the very real possibility of the complete medicalization and commodification of all phases of human procreation and birth.

Yet the description of the medical technologies as an attack on women, which for a number of feminist critics is signaled by sex-predetermination and sex-preselection technologies that could eliminate the female as a group before birth, does not fully capture the forces that propel this industrialization of life. To understand the advance of technologies that appear to give individual women precise knowledge of their efforts to achieve or maintain healthy pregnancies, we must turn again to the long-term historical and cultural forces which valorize predictability, control, and scientific evidence. Once again, we face a central paradox of contemporary feminism that this book has been naming. Though some feminists have raised profound questions about the new reproductive technologies, the liberatory ideal of freedom through control of fertility that feminism proclaims is intimately entwined with the modern worldview that the phenomena of the human and the natural world are proper objects for the exercise of human manipulation.

It is for this reason that many feminists view technologies which promise maximum individual choice and control over the timing of reproductive decisions and the "products" of pregnancy as enhancing women's freedom. For example, some of the most vociferous critics of the harm and danger of the new technologies have at the same time argued for access to artificial insemination. The distinction typically made is that, as a technical procedure, artificial insemination does not necessitate reliance on the high-tech medical establishment.[18] While those who are most critical of the medicalization of women's lives draw the line at artificial insemination, for feminist who are primarily interested in establishing the rights of procreation and child-rearing for individuals who do not fit within traditional definitions of the family, the crucial issue is equal access to technological advances. In the latter view, "If reproductive technology makes it possible for an unmarried person to have her or his own child, it is discriminatory and socially unwise to deny that person the right to procreate simply because she or he may be unable to find a suitable spouse, be unwilling to marry, or objects to heterosexual intercourse."[19] That is, in a world where everything "should" be manipulated to serve human happiness, rights become the mechanism for eradicating all barriers to the technologically feasible. This vision of individual freedom through technological modes of (re)production is an expression of the commodity logic of our society.

Surveillance and Population Control

We might imagine that ecologists who often define the problem of the contemporary world as one of "overpopulation" would be critical of the new reproductive technologies that facilitate birth. But this is not necessarily the case. Here again the modern managerial ethic, which originally provided a political language for the concept of a "population," has become intrinsic to mainstream ecological movements.

For many in these movements, prenatal selection technologies are especially appealing as a means of limiting family size. Such technologies may be utilized in the third world as a mechanism to reduce the birth rate, for instance. With the ability to "plan" births through amniocentesis and the subsequent abortion of female fetuses, couples in countries such as China may no longer "keep trying" to get a highly desired son. For others, emergent sex-determination technologies, in which women's ovulatory cycles are manipulated so as to maximize successful conception through the insertion of seminal fluid where the proportion of y chromosomes has been artificially increased, are preferable to sex-selection through abortion. In some scenarios, the birth of far more boys than girls would reduce the population because there would be fewer women to bear children.[20] Of course none of this population logic asks what the artificial reduction of the number of female children means for the status and well-being of women. In any case, the appeal of genetic screening as a mechanism of population control is considerably more complicated than the manipulation of sex ratios.

Concern about size of populations has been linked to concern about the quality of populations since the second half of the nineteenth century. In the late 1960s this linkage resurfaced with the new focus on the population explosion. This concern is found across the spectrum of politics. Whereas radical ecologists who belong to Earth First! may proclaim "Love your mother, don't become one," other patriarchal population control advocates who are less critical of reductionist science than typical Earth Firsters are fond of the use of the use of sex preselection technologies. The Secretary of the American Eugenics society argued that "American Society, if it takes its responsibility to future generations seriously, will have to do more than control the size of its population . . . [it] will have to take steps to insure that individuals yet unborn will have the best genetic and environmental heritage possible."[21] In 1971 the retiring president of the American Association for the Advancement of Science focused again on the language of rights, stating that:

> In a world where each pair must be limited on the average to two offspring and no more, the right that must become paramount is . . . the right of every child to be born with a sound physical and mental constitution, based on a sound genotype. No parents will in that future time have a right to burden society with a malformed or a mentally incompetent child. . . . Every child has the inalienable right to a sound heritage.[22]

By the 1980s the focus had shifted to fetal rights, even among scholars who supported a woman's right to choose abortion. Thus in 1983 a professor of law writes about the obligations a mother incurs once she chooses not to abort:

> These obligations may require her to avoid work, recreation, and medical care choices that are hazardous to the fetus. They also obligate her to preserve her health for the fetus's sake or even allow established therapies to be performed on an affected fetus. Finally, they require that she undergo prenatal screening where there is reason to believe that this screening may identify congenital defects correctable with available therapies.[23]

Whereas eugenics traditionally advocated (and continues to do so) the sterilization of "the feebleminded" and those of "inferior" races, today the notion of the right of a child to be born healthy, grounded in the new ability to monitor "health" before birth, has begun to replace overt eugenics. The possibilities of monitoring are suggested in a manual for physicians and genetic counselors from the late 1980s where the author argues, "genetic counseling is best offered routinely and systematically prior to marriage."[24] Medical records, prescriptive literature and consumer education that permeate the entire society are used to monitor the "correct" behavior of all pregnant women throughout the course of pregnancy. A pregnant woman is said to have the duty to insure that the fetus in her body "is born with sound mind and body."[25] Ads by organizations such as the American Cancer Society have cast cigarette smoking by pregnant women as a form of child abuse.[26] And on the issue of alcohol, while no labels warn the general population about the possibility of alcoholism, the proscriptions regarding alcohol and pregnancy are extensive. Under the new regime of safe pregnancy, a pregnant woman who likes an occasional drink to help her relax is now a pariah, a "bad" mother. One might well argue that today's "quality" control is maintained through a variety of apparatuses that shape, reshape, and mold the behavior and desires of all potentially pregnant women. Women who deviate from accepted norms may find themselves socially ostracized, but they may also find themselves "corrected" by the traditional arm of law. Cynthia Daniels reports that "by 1992, one hundred and sixty-seven pregnant women had been criminally prosecuted for delivering drugs to the fetus through the umbilical cord, for prenatal child neglect or abuse (for consuming alcohol or drugs during pregnancy), or for manslaughter in cases where a pregnancy ended in the delivery of a stillborn baby."[27] Hospital authorities have obtained court orders to mandate Cesarean deliveries (which are more common today because of the information produced by the now routine electronic fetal monitors) for women who do not want them but whose doctors deem that they are necessary. Women have also been forced to obtain maternal blood transfusions, or fetal medical treatments like intrauterine transfusions. Women have been prosecuted for failing to follow doctor's orders regarding sexual practices during pregnancy. And two weeks after the legalization of Norplant, Darlene Johnson, a twenty-eight year -old unwed mother on Welfare who was convicted of child abuse, was ordered to have Norplant implanted as a condition of parole.[28] Not surprisingly, poor women and women of color are more likely to find themselves the subjects of criminal prosecution. Marlene Garber Fried and Loretta Ross report that all of the drug and alcohol prosecutions to date have been of low-income women, of which more than 70 percent have been black women.[29]

A range of feminists from differing political positions have been outraged by this most recent effort to use the law to advance racist goals. In thinking about how to respond, we cannot fail to take account of the extent to which eugenics is back in fashion. As John Horgan notes in a powerful critique of the dubious links between genes and behavior in the June 1993 issue of *Scientific American*,

> The message that genetics can explain, predict and even modify human behavior for the betterment of society is promulgated not just on sensationalistic talk shows but by our prominent scientists. James D. Watson, co-discoverer of the double-helix structure of DNA and former head of the Human Genome Project, the massive effort to map our entire genetic endowment, said recently, "We used to think that our fate was in our stars. Now we know, in large part, that our fate is in our genes."[30]

Ecofeminism and New Reproductive Technologies

The unrestrained manipulation of procreation and birth can move too easily from the lending of a helping hand to the production of human beings on specification. And I am very queasy about how we measure the success of our assorted interventions. The birth of an apparently healthy baby is surely very tangible, but what about the fate of that baby through the course of her life? The scientific profession's short-term focus on "product" takes little account of the long-term consequences of actions which maximize control today. As the biochemist Irwin Chargaff warns, "In manipulating processes worked out by nature in the wisdom of millions of years one must be aware of the dangers that our shortcuts may carry a bleeding edge."[31] The systematic elimination of genes from the human gene pool that are deemed undesirable and unproductive today—in effect an effort to reduce diversity and homogenize life—may over the course of generations prove to be disastrously short-sighted and imprudent. We already know that the effort to perfect the seeds that generate food has severely reduced the diversity that sustains agricultural abundance, making crops vulnerable to pestilence and blight in ways that are totally unprecedented.

These are issues that are constantly on my mind. Yet after a new marriage, a miscarriage, and a diagnosis of fibroids, I found that I, too, wanted doctors and machines to provide answers and assurances. When I did get pregnant one doctor told me that it could be difficult, that they might have to decide to go in and get the baby out early, but I should be encouraged because the local hospital was doing a good job of keeping premature babies alive after only six months' gestation. I felt pretty certain that I would never consent to such a scenario, but in discussing the issues with my husband, who was deeply drawn to the possibility of having a child, I began to wonder about the difference between saving a fetus and more routine operations for a sick child. After miscarrying again, and becoming pregnant once more, my deep reservations about sonograms faded. I felt I needed to know if this third fetus was still alive. I agonized about what to do about amniocentesis, but decided to at least go through the standard counseling process to see what it was all about from the inside. When I explained some of my reservations, that I felt it was akin to trying to play God, the genetics counselor quickly responded that counseling did not deal with "morals." I asked why the recommended age for amniocentesis in my city was now thirty-four, and she confessed that she thought it was because of the greater availability of services. Yet she agreed that such availability might not be the best reason to recommend the procedure. I left feeling pretty confident and strong; I had seen how the system operated and I felt I could resist. Even though I was the "advanced" age of forty-one and would have to endure bewildered queries from family and friends, I was going to accept "risks." After all, my mother had given birth to me when she was my age. She didn't know what all the fuss about tests was all about.

But after I miscarried and became pregnant again, I was six months older and found in more difficult to dismiss the numbers that seemed to be stacked against me. Whereas earlier I had concentrated on the risks of the procedure itself and thought how silly it would be to endanger a pregnancy I had been hoping for for two years, now I began to admit to myself that at my age with two grown children, my desire for a child might not be strong enough to care for one with special needs. I was beginning to struggle with these new thoughts, when the doctor asked again about amnio. By this time we had our prepared response, but the doctor's paternal advice about what *his* wife would do, in the midst of my own doubts, left me emotionally vulnerable and confused. The tests now seemed reassuring if not necessary. Yet how could I live with myself given my condemnations of the system? I finally decided I could go ahead because my criticisms concerned the routinization of screening, not the technology per se. The "system" wouldn't sustain itself if it only had the business of women my age.

When the day for my amnio finally arrived I was feeling pretty good physically. I assumed my bouts of morning sickness and just plain sickness had passed because I had gotten past the difficult first trimester. The initial sonogram showed, however, that I was no longer pregnant—the fetus had died. In our initial shock and despair, it was somehow comforting to hear the geneticist tell me and my husband that given the three losses, it would now be appropriate to test our genes for a transposed chromosome. If this were the case, my chance of giving birth to a normal baby was low, but even then, we were told, we shouldn't be discouraged because with proper checking they had gotten other people successfully through pregnancies. On the way home as I took note of my feelings, I thought "How could I ever criticize a woman who chose in-vitro fertilization?"

When I got home I realized that what the doctor had meant by "checking" was chorionic villi sampling, a diagnostic chromosome procedure similar to amniocentesis that can be done as early as eight weeks rather than the fifteen weeks for amnio. I knew that the test was still considered experimental in some places, but now I realized that if I became pregnant again, I might actually "choose" the less tested procedure to provide what I thought of as protection against another second-trimester miscarriage. I would want to know earlier that the pregnancy was doomed. Yet, I also realized that in a very real sense I had been blessed. What if the fetus had not died and I had the amnio and been told that the chromosomes were not "normal"? Just that afternoon I had seen two children: a teenager in a wheelchair unable to hold his head up while being fed by his mother, and a young boy about twelve, who had that angelic look that some Downs Syndrome children have, walking along very zestfully with an older brother or friend. Those two images within a half-hour of each other were a vivid reminder that prenatal testing does not tell how severe a child's problems will be. I had been spared from having to make a decision about life with a diagnostic category that did not distinguish between these children.

As the days passed, I became obsessed with trying to determine if our problems were a result of my husband's working in a nuclear submarine plant as a teenager and spending many summers swimming in the bay that adjoined the plant. (The knowledge that a childhood friend of his who had also lived in the same city had given birth to a baby with cancer spurred our concern.) Upon mentioning this concern to the counselor, I received a prompt call from the geneticist who wanted to assure me that there was no relationship between our problems now and whatever radiation exposure my husband may have had as a youth.[32] But when the diagnostic test we were waiting for was completed, there was initial confusion. My name had been accidentally placed on the vial with my husband's blood sample. Although the test had been negative, because of the mislabeling the lab technicians thought the sample had been contaminated since they had found male chromosomes in "female" blood. When they discovered what had happened, they offered me a free test. (Since the initial hypothesis was that my husband had a transposed chromosome, only his blood had been sampled, and the test showed that this was not the case.) It was assumed we would avail ourselves of this opportunity. But by this time, I found the strength and perspective to say "no." Our glimpse into the system's problems and mistakes helped us to realize that the information that this seductive science could produce was not likely to lead to birth or the wisdom we needed to cope with the uncertainties we faced.

When I suddenly found myself pregnant again a little less than a year later I did decide to do the chorionic villi sampling at eight weeks, and, other than much amusement that we had to pay an extra fee not to be told the sex of the fetus, my experiences of new technologies this time around were rather positive. I marveled as my older obstetrician who had scandalized the medical community by turning babies around in utero so a Cesarean could be avoided used a sonogram monitor to guide his hands to shift this fetus away from a breech position seven months into the pregnancy. The best of the new and the best of the old I thought! My older body however was not as supple as it had been nineteen years earlier. My eyes were so tightly closed as I scrunched my body to push that I didn't even see a baby fall out. Told I had just delivered a baby girl I fell into a state of wonder.

My own negotiation through the world of baby-making (which did not include clinics and lawyers' offices where alternative conception technologies are sometimes pursued) has impressed on me once again that there are no straight forward answers for individual women. I have no illusions that an ecological perspective will somehow eliminate the pain of infertility, immediately solve the dilemmas of lesbian or gay partners who want to parent, or the anxiety pregnant mothers have for the health of their children. Nonetheless, after my own venture into the world of reproductive technologies, I am more convinced than ever of our need for an ethic of interconnectedness very different from the instrumental ethic dominant in Western, particularly American, culture which assumes the vulnerabilities of the body can be conquered.

This dominant masculinist ethic dissects fertility and human reproduction, with the explicit goal of improving the operation of the reproductive system's parts. An alternative ethic of interconnectedness would take heed of the intricate links between the birth and well-being of all animals—human as well as nonhuman—with the preservation of the earth's ecosystems.[33] In a fragmented culture that is ambivalent and fearful about women's bodies, where the language of liberation is wedded to entities with rights, and where the dominant culture increasingly stresses the importance of "a child with one's own genes," it is tremendously difficult to comprehend these ecosystemic and social webs, even those which are intuitively reasonable. Yet try we must. Otherwise, we face the homogenization and control of all life on Earth.

FOOD
WITHOUT SWEAT:
FROM
ABUNDANCE
FOR ALL
TO THE
POISONING
OF THE PLANET

Soldiers spray the largest "enemies" with bullets, agriculturalists spray the smallest "enemies" with their chemical solutions. . . . Spray an enemy people's soldiers to death and an indispensable part of the human family has been subjected to a treatment the consequences of which no one can estimate. Spray the parasites of the grapevines and one destroys the life in the earth under which the grapevine cannot live.

ELIN WAGNER,
Alarmclock

❧

Pity the nation that wears a cloth it does not weave, eats a bread it does not harvest, and drinks a wine that flows not from its own wine press.

KHALIL GIBRAN,
The Prophet

❧

In the traditional economy, time was plentiful and limited only by the course of the seasons. . . . The Ladakhis now have less time . . . they are losing their once-acute sensitivity to the nuances of the world around them—the ability, for instance, to detect the slightest variations in the weather, or in the movement in the stars. A friend from the Markha Valley summed it up for me: "I can't understand it. My sister in the capital, she now has all these things that do the work faster. She just buys her clothes in a shop, she has a jeep, a telephone, a gas cooker. All of these things save so much time, and yet when I go to visit her, she doesn't have time to talk with me."

HELENA NORBERG-HODGE,
Ancient Futures: Learning from Ladakh

ALDOUS HUXLEY'S *BRAVE NEW WORLD*, WRITTEN in 1931, painted a sterile dystopia where punishment was rare, but thoroughgoing control was exercised through genetic standardization and the manipulation of rewards. As a teenager growing up in the early sixties I was fascinated and disconcerted by Huxley's view of the possibilities of rationality, most especially his depiction of the mechanized control of baby production. But it wasn't until my feminism began to be reshaped by ecological consciousness that I realized the total industrialization of life, so vividly portrayed by Huxley, could not be fully appreciated with a lens focused only on human bodies.

As we saw in the last chapter, the contemporary "advances" in reproductive technology seem to move us closer to a "brave new world." The mechanization and standardization of human procreation and birth, from bedside computerized charting of fertility cycles to maximize the chances of conception, to clinical gamete-intrafallopian transfer, prenatal selection of desirable fetuses, and emergent sex-determination technologies, is a powerful demonstration of our seemingly endless drive to eradicate the mysterious and contain the unpredictable. Disturbing as these developments are, they take on a different cast when viewed in the context of the increasing level of assaults on the fertility of the earth.

Huxley also deplored assaults on the earth, but what is most vexing about Huxley's prescient vision is that his critique of the dominant form of rationality did not inform his understanding of ecological questions. For Huxley, like Paul Ehrlich, Garret Hardin, and the other more ecologically minded new-Malthusians who were to shortly follow, "the problem of rapidly increasing numbers in relation to natural resources . . . is now the central problem of mankind."[1] This insistence that the problem is numbers brings us to Thomas Malthus again and his dire warning in 1798 of a perpetual scarcity of food. Malthus argued that food production was incapable of meeting the demands of too many human mouths in industrializing England. In our contemporary world, the concern is more typically the issue of adequate food production in postcolonial nations. What I find most important in understanding the overpopulation debate is not the strengths or weaknesses of the methods used to project numbers. Rather, I want to look at how the fear of too many people is linked with a narrative of progress in which scarcity is defeated by newfound technological abundance. It is this narrative of control that must be contested if the modern assault on the earth is to be effectively resisted. Moreover, in taking up this challenge we must also take account of how this fear of numbers (which for many is inextricably linked to dark bodies) is produced by graphic images that portray the imagined horrors of overcrowding and a youthful population reproducing itself.

The Production of Abundance

For the contemporary essayist Wendell Berry, who is also a farmer in rural Kentucky, one of the more debilitating effects of the narrative of progress is its "colonization of the future," a morally questionable process that facilitates the poisoning of the earth. Berry's analysis, focussed primarily on the United States, is especially sensitive to how the projection of the future, and the all-purpose threat of starvation, has been used to industrialize food production: "The most prolific source of justification for exploitative behavior has been the future. . . . The future is a time that cannot be reached except by industrial progress and economic growth. The future, so full of material blessings, is nevertheless threatened with dire shortages of food energy, and security unless we exploit the earth even more 'freely,' with greater speed and less caution."[2] In this possible future, potential scarcity looms vividly in a world deprived of technological wonders, resembling earlier societies (primitive, tribal, uncivilized, pagan) which are said to be heavily marked by want and despair. But if we refuse to accept this view's insistence that scarcity is the universal human condition, the world that comes into view may take on decidedly different characteristics. Whether the leisure and ready availability of food in many hunter gatherer societies made them the "original affluent society," whether medieval peasants really had over 150 holidays a year, or whether West Coast Native Americans really only "worked" three hours a day, newer ethnographic and historical interpretations strongly argue against positing deprivation as a general human condition.[3]

Alternative readings of the human situation on Earth suggest that scarcity—as opposed to periods of insufficiency—was invented with the birth of consumer society in eighteenth century Europe. As Nicholas Xenos provocatively notes,

> Once the experience of scarcity took hold in modernity, abundance took shape as the ideal negation of the present order. . . . Eventually, the concept of progress provided a narrative structure within which scarcity and abundance could be accommodated in a single linear frame. Scarcity could then be cast as the antagonist in the human story, a story with a happy ending; the vanquishing of the antagonist and a life of happiness ever after amid abundance for all.[4]

This narrative of progress as happiness has proven to be extremely resilient, despite the wars, ecological havoc, and social disruptions that have been its underside. It has been the principle means by which non-Western stories and forms of knowledge have been marginalized and made irrelevant to the course of Western history.[5]

In the contemporary period, this narrative of progress which shaped the emergence of consumer society in the West has been invoked within a new discourse that circumscribes the planet itself. Under the discourse of "development," abundance is to be extended to all residents of the planet through the fruits of scientific knowledge that have accumulated in the West. This move to extend the powers of modern science to all corners of the globe has been traced to President Harry Truman's inaugural address of January of 1949 in which he called for "a bold new program for making the benefits of our scientific advances and industrial progress available for improvement and growth of underdeveloped areas." As Mexican writer Gustave Esteva notes, "In an instant two billion people became 'underdeveloped,' stripped of their dignity and the richness of their cultural diversity, homogenized and redefined in terms of what they were not."[6] Whereas Foucault had identified the barracks, schools, hospitals, and prisons as the places where the disciplining of human bodies for social improvement took place in modernizing Europe, today the developing nations of the world are the new setting for those various techniques of power which seek to integrate the most marginalized regions and groups into the benefits of technological and educational modernization, improving their everyday skills and habits and producing "abundance" for all.

The "out of control" growth of indigenous populations is often blamed for our environmental crises. Whether it is the decimated forests of India, the unbreathable air in contemporary Jakarta, or the undrinkable water of Bombay, the notion of "burgeoning populations" is typically invoked as the self-evident explanation for why the Earth is not well. This explanation is crudely reductionist, but what is wrong with today's development enterprise and its promise of a better life cannot be fully appreciated without taking a closer look at the technologies of power that have produced material abundance in the West.

In the introduction to this book I suggested that the dream of food without sweat is one of the enticements by which disciplinary power advances. This dream of harvesting the riches of the Earth without having to be reminded of our bodies, a dream of pleasure without toil, harkens back to the garden of Eden. This alluring utopian fantasy was dramatically transformed into a palpable possibility for large numbers of people with the complicated social changes wrought by the end of feudalism, the advent of colonialism, and the scientific revolution of the seventeenth century. The enclosure of the commons, the development of capitalist modes of production, and the movement away from the land in the following centuries created societies whose dependence on the land was disguised and obscured. By the nineteenth century, the social and physical nature of work which sustains daily life was even further obscured.

In the twentieth century, advances in the mechanization of agriculture, the application of petrochemicals, the harnessing of the Earth's waters, the development of hybrid seeds, the breeding of vegetables for harvesting and processing specifications, the development of total confinement buildings for farm animals, and the routinized use of antibiotics, medicated feed, and hormonal growth stimulants, together with advances in energy-intensive processing, transportation, and refrigeration have created a situation in which our food, formerly the fruit of the Earth's fertility, has become yet another factory product. For all but a few of us in advanced industrialized countries, the links between the sustenance of our bodies and the sustenance from and of the Earth has been totally severed. Our bodies have become as Berry puts it, "a conduit which channels the nutrients of the earth to the sewer."[7] Fruits and vegetables are no longer a reminder of the cycles of the seasons, and the suffering and killing that produce meat are invisible. As the distance between farm and table has grown, the packaging that was deemed necessary for the production of sanitized food and the new standards of convenience has produced noxious garbage that cannot be returned to the Earth. The cycles of life have been so totally altered that even rain from the sky can be filled with man-made contaminants. Where animals on integrated farms had been participants in humus making, contributing to the replenishment of the soil, concentrated livestock production now produces "waste" that escapes into the air and into the waters as gaseous ammonia. In this new chain, the resultant acid soils and acid rains signaled a barren rather than a fertile future.[8]

From a world where both genders routinely interacted with the Earth, we have moved into a world where food is most often something that magically appears on men's tables. The movement in the mid-nineteenth century, for example, from homegrown and locally ground grains to mass-produced, superfine flours, which Ruth Schwartz Cowan documents, meant that men no longer participated in the hauling and milling of grain: "Men's share in domestic activity began to disappear, while women's increased."[9] The remaining reminders that food required toil, such as meal-planning, cooking, and cleaning became strictly the work of women. In a similar fashion the sanitized purification of the body afforded by flush toilets and water-borne sewage systems (which also pollute rivers and disrupt the fertility cycle of the Earth), did not fall equally on men's and women's bodies. Women became responsible for keeping new water closets clean, and modern water and utility systems meant that everything in the house had to be kept even cleaner.[10]

Material abundance had been created. But at what cost? For Wendell Berry, the new manufactured paradise has been produced by the "substitutions of energy for knowledge, of methodology for care, of technology for morality."[11] The consequences for the land and people have been ruinous. The yields of the new heavily researched hybrid strains (corn, wheat, sorghum) were so spectacular that they were often referred to as "miracle crops." Yet these large fields of miracle crops are totally lacking in genetic diversity, making them extremely vulnerable to insects and disease and requiring greater and greater amounts of deadly chemical pesticides.[12]

Synthetic pesticides were the commercial outgrowth of World War II chemical warfare research, just as the technology that produced bombs was used after the war to produce the nitrogen fertilizers that the new high yield crops required. Unfortunately these new petrochemical fertilizers were also implicated in the destruction of the earth's ozone layer. The macabre connections between war and the methods of the new agripower are not simple. Fertilizers after World War II were so productive that they also encouraged weeds, which under the prevailing logic required herbicides. Since herbicides sometimes killed crops too, the call for genetically engineered plants that would be herbicide resistant intensified. During the Vietnam War, herbicides decimated forests, rubber plantations, and rice paddies, leaving whole sections of the Earth dead and institutionalizing ecocide as an integral part of U.S. military policy.[13]

Agricultural technology, developed in universities and multinational seed, chemical, and biotechnology institutes—in its everyday ordinariness of extracting more than it returns—is integral to the contemporary "laboratory" state, effecting a mode of warfare more insidious than the traditional horror of battle. The scale of the Earth's poisoning—the loss of genetic diversity, the depletion and erosion of soil, the pollution of lakes, rivers, and oceans by the runoff of contaminated topsoil, the destruction of underground aquifers from pollution and overuse, the damage to the air, and the poisoning of the food chain itself—is staggering.

It is crucial to note that this routine destruction of the Earth proceeds, not through the traditional martial powers of generals and kings, but through the enticement of material abundance and the dream of realizing food without sweat. In the global context this dream of progress, shaped as it is by the narrative of scarcity to abundance, has permitted U.S. agripower to deem indigenous forms of knowledge thoroughly deficient and inferior.

Fertility and Colonialism

> When we burn grass for grasshoppers, we don't ruin things.
> We shake down acorns and pinenuts. But the White people
> plow up the ground, pull down the trees, kill everything. . . .
> They blast rocks and scatter them on the ground. . . . How
> can the spirit of the earth like the White man? . . .
> Everywhere the White man has touched it, it is sore.
>   WINTU WOMAN, CALIFORNIA, FROM *Touch the Earth*

In accounting for the material abundance of the industrialized West it is important to take note that the West has few genetic riches in comparison to other areas of the globe. The West's abundance was fueled by colonial interventions in the food production of colonies and the seizure of the botanical treasures of the tropics and subtropics. In the mid-eighteenth century, for example, the number of exotic flora entering the British Isles to supply the gardens and greenhouses of the aristocracy increased ninefold. Cary Fowler and Pat Mooney argue that "To an extent which has not been properly recognized, the history of colonialism is a history of the struggle to capture and monopolize botanical treasurers."[14] The general pattern was one of the uprooting of crops from one continent to another, combined with enforced cash crop production for metropolitan countries. In West Africa, for example, colonial administrations imposed on local farmers monocultures of annual crops for export. Cotton was produced to supply British and French textile mills. This pattern of growing the same crops year after year on the same land without the traditional mixing of crops, trees, and livestock rapidly robbed the soil of its fertility. In many places Europeans seized the most fertile and well-watered lands for themselves. Societies that had had food in abundance were thus introduced to scarcity and malnutrition. The comments of a French colonial inspector on a mission to famine-stricken Upper Volta in 1932 are noteworthy in this regard: "One can only wonder how it happens that . . . people, once accustomed to food abundance are now living from hand to mouth. . . . I feel morally bound to point out that the intensification of the policy of giving priority to industrial products has coincided with an increase in the frequency of food shortages."[15] Self-provisioning communities were transformed into export enclaves through forced commercialization and the introduction of private property in land. Land that was not cultivated was deemed wasteland. Forests were thus clearfelled as a way of turning "waste" into the wealth of cultivated land. In the latter part of the nineteenth century, when the British recognized the revenue-generating capacity of Indian forests, protecting the forests was defined as denying villagers access to them as a common resource.

These processes of mining the Earth impoverished large numbers of both men and women, but women tended to suffer more. The imposition of export crop production by European agricultural agents, who were accustomed to dealing with men and male farming systems, made women's historic role as food-producers peripheral wherever colonialism traveled. In general, with the introduction of private property, women lost customary use rights and inheritance rights to land.[16]

Colonization operated on both ideological and material levels. British colonization of Indian forests, for example fractured the symbolic goddess imagery that expressed the indigenous culture's veneration of the forest as the highest expression of the earth's fertility. At the material level, subsistence economies—in which the forest was both sacred and multifunctional, supplying food, fuel, fodder, fertilizer, fiber, and medicine—were displaced by what Vandana Shiva terms the "one dimensional, masculinist science of forestry."[17] Though the particular spiritual beliefs differed from place to place, the general pattern of colonization, from the original European conquest of North and South America to the subsequent conquest of the entire globe, was the delegitimation of beliefs that honored the earth as the giver of life. As Shiva puts it, "throughout the world, the colonization of diverse peoples was, at its root, a forced subjugation of ecological concepts of nature."[18] Instead of complex rituals, oral traditions, and farming practices that cultivated the interdependence of humans with the fertility of the Earth, the Earth was rendered into an object totally distinct from the autonomous human self. In this process of separating humans from the world around, sensuous relations between human and animal were criminalized and the erotic became more fully human centered.[19] The earth's only purpose was to produce resources, primarily for the humans in the colonial nations.

The Introduction of Development

John S. Aird, a former senior research specialist on China at the U.S. Bureau of the Census, has observed that

[the idea of a "population crisis"] ascribes many of the world's ills—including poverty, hunger, health problems, housing shortages, transportation problems, illiteracy,

✳ lack of education, unemployment, overcrowding, resource
depletion, soil erosion, and environmental degradation—to
a single factor, prescribes a single remedy, and invests the
combination with a sense of great certitude. . . . It is the sort
of cause that inspires zeal. For governments in developing
countries, the population crisis idea has the added virtue of
putting the blame for socioeconomic problems on the reproductive habits of the people rather than on defective
political leadership or misconceived policies.[20]

In the post World War II era, "development" was introduced as a postcolonial project that would presumably not
entail the subjugation and exploitation that had occurred in
previous eras. Rather, previously colonized places entered
into the policies of industrial nations in two distinct yet intimately related ways. The first was to construe third world
peoples as "populations." Today this eighteenth century
construction of humans living together is so completely
accepted that all parties to population debates, whatever
their ideological persuasion, assume that populations are
constitutive of reality. But as Foucault notes in his *History
of Sexuality*:

> One of the great innovations in the techniques of power in the
> eighteenth century was the emergence of "population" as an
> economic and political problem: population as wealth, popu-
> lation as manpower or labor capacity, population balanced
> between its growth and the resources it commanded. Govern-
> ments perceived that they were not simply dealing with the
> subjects, or even with a "people," but with a population.[21]

With the spread of quantitative reasoning and statistics, the
belief developed "that people can be managed just as dependent variables can be controlled."[22] Since the granting of
independence to former colonies, an incessant fear has been
that if too many of "them" propagate, the ability of Western industrialized nations to maintain their level of con-

sumption will be severely threatened. In this view the material well-being of the West depends upon the continued bounty of the entire earth, a bounty which could be compromised by the fertility and reproduction of previously colonized third world peoples. At the same time, the ceaseless claims of overpopulation are countered by the claims about improving the fertility of the soil. The propaganda of the "Green revolution" has held out the promise of extending abundance in third as well as first world nations. In this case fertility is not being controlled to limit family size, but rather enhanced by agricultural technologies. A further paradox of the promise of the Green revolution is that loans and technology which were held out to equalize wealth and productive capacity in Africa, Latin America, and Asia have forged complicated new bonds of dependence and poverty, in many cases arguably deeper and more problematic than the situation they were meant to alleviate.

As I suggested earlier the allure of food, health, and material goods for all, including those in desperately impoverished countries, belies the institutional practices that are implemented to achieve those ideals. These practices lead to abuse, poisoning, and depletion of the Earth's riches. Now, new national elites rather than colonial powers have masterminded the exploitation of indigenous peoples. One of the more egregious symbols of the science/commercialization nexus is the well known case of Western companies promoting baby formula with free samples in areas where women lacked both the cash to obtain sufficient supplies and access to clean water. In addition to increased infant mortality and malnutrition, the decline in breastfeeding meant the fertility of fewer women was being naturally regulated, which under the prevailing logic created the need for more efficient technological modes of contraception.

Marxist analyses have been very important in illuminating the material interests that have been served by colonialist and more recent imperialist practices. Yet because the

Marxist dream is itself propelled by the promise of abundance, it is insufficiently attentive to the complex mechanisms of enticement by which the dream of food without sweat is extended to all corners of the globe. Media satellites beam prescribed visions of the good life through an array of channels that defy the imagination. The opening of a McDonalds or a western style medical clinic, for example, is typically greeted with great enthusiasm in communities that previously did not have access to such "opportunities." Wangari Maathai of the Kenyan Green Belt movement bemoans how highly refined foods like bread and tinned vegetables are now considered signs of affluence and progress.[23] In Indonesia, as in so many parts of the world, lands harboring nutritionally important wild plants such as gnetum, sauropus, and hibiscus manihot are converted to the domestic production of fashionable imported vegetables like cauliflower, carrots, and cucumbers.[24] In each instance imperial signs of abundance become the objects of desire in postcolonial cultures, desires that cannot be met without increased environmental destruction and social stratification.

The abundance of the West is still fueled by harnessing the sweat and biological riches of the poorer nations. Today the mining of plants and human labor takes place at the most microlevels of life, as biotech companies of the North utilize the germ plasm of the South to produce new industrial products that can then be resold at handsome profits to food-producers across the globe.[25] In the contemporary era, though, the pursuit of material abundance has been so destructive of the biological diversity sustaining abundance that the fates of both rich and poor nations have become intertwined.

Today, policymakers and political leaders who have very little sense of a living Earth, nevertheless still speak of "our common future" and thus feel compelled to send negotiators and managers to gatherings such as the 1992 Earth Summit. Our common future may not be a beneficent one. The pillaging of rainforests in the South cannot be isolated from the climactic changes that are affecting all life on the planet. The Earth is losing topsoil at a pace that threatens food production across the globe. The loss of diversity threatens life itself. One might hope that this emergent awareness of interdependence and the fragility of the Earth's ecosystems would lead to serious questioning of the present pursuit of abundance, opening up a strategy of "de-development" among the overconsumers of the North. But as the Centre for Science and Environment warns in a 1991 report on global warming, the contemporary focus on environmental concerns seems to be leading to a new form of colonialism, an environmental colonialism in which data on greenhouse gas emissions are manipulated to support the idea that the developing world must share the blame for heating up the Earth. This idea can then be used to thrust even greater degrees of global discipline on already subjugated nations.[26] Thus both pro- and antidevelopment forces come together in response to the North's efforts to police and monitor the practices of the South. Where the former feel it is simply unjust for the North to tell the South they should be deprived of the benefits of industrialization, the latter focuses on the need for the North to change its consumption patters. Not surprisingly, the new concern with environmental matters opens different paths for reconstruction, a subject that I will return to in the next chapter.

Women and Development

The German sociologist Maria Mies' interview with a woman from Kunur, a rural Indian village, illuminates some of the gender dynamics of the social stratification that has accompanied the introduction of development and the modernization of agriculture:

Q. How long have you been here?
A. Since the time of the birth of this village. But now,

after the current (electricity) has come, our life has been difficult. Earlier our men used to go to pull water from the irrigation canals in the fields. Now they (the Doras) have motors. We are no longer required. They felt that our wage is an extra expense for them and why should they pay us unnecessarily. That money they can save and take home. Even their women feel that most of their profit is wasted on wages. Therefore, they ask their men to do the little bit of work in the fields themselves and save the money. Because of them we are unable to live. It was like that since they got this current. Earlier it was better. We used to get all the food grain we needed for our work. Now we do not get anything.

Q. Why not?

A. Due to this current. Now they have motor pumps. Before nothing could move without us. They needed us for all work in the fields. Now is is not like that. Because of their motor pumps they can do everything themselves. When they need us, they call us, but when they do not need us, they do not call. When one of their animals dies, they call us to remove the corpse. Formerly we sued to get grain and 2 rupees for kallu (country liquor) when we removed the dead body. Now they give us only 10 rupees and they also give it to us as if they were doing us a favor, not our due wage. This we get only once in a while.[27]

The depletion of the fertility of the "skin of the Earth," the ravaging of her forests, the despoliation of her air, and the pollution of her waters is not specific to the South, but, as an ecofeminist perspective makes clear, it is women of the South who are bearing the brunt of destructive processes.

With the launching of the U.N. Decade for Women in 1975 a new object of attention was identified in the offices of the World Bank, U.S.A.I.D. and the other institutions of the dense international development apparatus—"women and development." Ester Boserup's enormously influential 1971 text, *Women's Role in Economic Development*, shaped a vast organizational infrastructure that insisted women's experience of development was not the same as that of men. With the data and testimony generated by the U.N.'s focus on women, and the demographic research indicating that enhancing women's status was an important key in reducing fertility rates, the discovery of "women" afforded a new opportunity for development specialists and population controllers to ply their trades. Integrating women more fully into the process of development and improving their relative status to men became an institutionalized concern in the development community and the human development and educational agencies of nations of the South. Projects designated as meeting the goals of women and development afforded yet another mechanism—one particularly suited to the concerns of today's world—for harnessing the energies of third world peoples. Pam Simmons suggests that the call to integrate women into development "was a whole new lease on life for the flagging development establishment."[28]

In the context of the contemporary global economy, the new focus on women and development made it possible to speak of woman as laborer (in contradistinction to population discourse, which spoke of woman only as a reproductive machine), thereby creating new subjects who could be integrated into the international cash economy. For the apostles of modernization, the production by women of handicrafts and small electronics for consumption in the West became a sign of progress, while also producing handsome profits for multinational corporations. The creation of income generation projects for women that would teach marketable skills became a popular mode of intervention for both development and population experts. Though the different training and educational projects rarely altered the social or economic power of the vast majority of all women in the South, for population controllers, the projects provided a convenient new tool for introducing a new norm that of the happy nuclear family with the designated number of two children. In Indonesia, for example, the UNFPA provided funds to women's groups to set up beekeeping, vegetable-raising, and handicraft businesses when women agreed to have only two children. Media images and educational materials throughout the South were deployed so as to suggest that "smaller families are happier families." Pictorial representations typically laid out the message that small families were smiling because their new contraceptive practices had permitted them to enter the world of ever increasing access to consumer goods. Traditionally this was taken to mean two children, but more recently, with all the attention given to China's one-child policies and the global focus on environmental degradation, India's family planners have sought to popularize the idea that happiness is one child. Today the happy nuclear family is depicted pushing a carriage with a single baby playing with a bountiful supply of toys.[29]

Yet the reconstitution of traditional joint households into consumer households is not merely a matter of demography. Consumer households may often indeed be smaller than traditional extended families. But at the same time the values and needs of these more "modern" and up-to-date familial arrangements (both those few that actually attain consumer status and the many that development has made destitute) typically result in a both a greater use of resources and increased environmental destruction. The prevailing population/development ideology is essentially incapable of dealing with this contradictory facet of its management plans because its calls for limiting population are based upon an underlying commitment to conventional growth economics. Thus, ironically, as the call for better and more thoroughgoing population control increases from all corners, the actual implementation of family planning expands the reign of scarcity and environmental degradation by absorbing ever more households into the global marketplace. (In January 1992 the chief health minister of India announced a new draft plan for family planning, declaring, "What we want is not more people but more things for people."[30]) In the pursuit of lifestyles of material abundance, joint households, who in caring for their kin pool their means of survival, and tend for soil, seeds, and water with an awareness of future generations, are relegated to the dustbins of history. Private nuclear families regulated by the state are an essential element of the new world order.

Until very recently the fact that the majority of women in the South are food-producers and that their ability to produce food and care for their households and the soil has been increasingly threatened by environmental destruction, was also ignored in discussions about women and development. But for analysts such as Bina Agarwal and Vandana Shiva, who were among the first to point to the new environmental threats to survival to women in developing countries like India, the burden of the disappearance of the forests of the South falls primarily on women and female children who must increase their labor in order to obtain water, fuelwood, and fodder.[31] Agarwal reports several cases of women committing suicide because their inability to obtain adequate supplies led to tensions with mothers-in-law in whose youth forests were plentiful.[32] Soil erosion and desertification, the literal drying up of the Earth's fertility (a result of deforestation as well as the marginalisation of women's traditional soil-building practices and the substitution of imported hybrid seeds for indigenous seeds conserved by women) has also made it more difficult for women to produce enough grain for sustenance. Women's work in producing food for survival is still necessary, but, as Shiva notes, their ability to do so has been weakened, "As more land is diverted to cash crops and is impoverished through the ecological impacts of the green revolution technologies, women have decreased space, but increased burdens in food production. With the market as the measure of all productivity, the 'value' of women's work and status falls, while their work in producing food for survival increases."[33]

Thus it is not surprising that it is largely in those regions where Green revolution technologies were the most systematically adopted that old sexist practices and traditions such as dowry intensified and new forms such as prenatal selection advanced. In India the introduction of wage labor—which has meant differential wage labor by sex—has led to increased dowry demands, which in turn has led to an increased demand for mechanisms that dispense with females. During a period when the official policy was to integrate women into development, fatal burnings of the bodies of young brides either through "accidents" or the collusion of angry in-laws and husbands became an everyday occurrence. And it was only after an error in an amniocentesis analysis resulted in the abortion of a male fetus that controversy arose over technologies which were promoted by advertisements promising, "Boy or girl of your choice." Amniocentesis for purposes of sex selection was available in rural areas where basic amenities like potable water and electricity did not exist. Rural health centers that did not have cold storage facilities for oral polio vaccine nonetheless routinely sent amniotic fluid in ice packs for analysis in Bombay.[34] The routinization of amniocentesis facilitated the systematic abortion of female fetuses.

The devaluation and hatred of women that is expressed in these prejudicial practices clearly did not originate with the Green revolution and amniocentesis. Dowry and female infanticide are ancient institutions. At the same time, the reductionist view of nature that is so entrenched in the West is a recent import into societies that have traditionally seen nature as a living being. For an ecofeminist (at least this one) the presence in such a society of practices that treat women as dispensable is profoundly troubling and requires detailed historical treatment that is beyond the scope of this book. But the fact that these misogynist practices have proliferated, rather than declined, in a period where development efforts are reputedly eliminating "backwardness," is additional evidence that development is linked to subjugation. The use to which amniocentesis has been put in India serves to buttress male power at the same time that it advances the concerns of population controllers seeking to fine-tune the fertility patterns of a "population." For specialists who comprehend the world through measurement, discarded female fetuses may be a negligible cost if fertility rates can be reduced through maximizing the birth of male children. Just as ecological consciousness is not intrinsic to feminism, feminist consciousness is not intrinsic to ecological thinking. It is not just any effort to save the Earth that will enhance the well-being of women.

OUR BODIES, OUR EARTH: THE POLITICS OF RENEWAL, RESTRUCTURING, AND RE-EVOLUTION

*In the most general sense of progressive thought, the Enlighten-
ment has always aimed at liberating men from fear and establishing their sovereignty. Yet the fully enlightened earth radiates disaster triumphant.*
MAX HORKHEIMER AND THEODORE W. ADORNO,
Dialectic of Enlightenment

*Throughout the world, a new questioning is growing, rooted in
the experience of those for whom the spread of what was called
"enlightenment" has been the spread of darkness, of the
extinction of life and life-enhancing processes.*
VANDANA SHIVA,
Staying Alive

*The continuing spiritual power of an image lives in the interplay
between what it reminds us of—what it brings to mind—and our
own continuing actions in the present. When the labrys becomes a
badge for a cult of Minoan goddesses, when the wearer of the
labrys has ceased to ask herself what she is doing on this earth,
where her love of women is taking her, the labrys, too becomes
abstraction—lifted away from the heat and friction of human
activity. The Jewish star on my neck must serve me both for
reminder and as a goad to continuing and changing responsibility.*
ADRIENNE RICH,
Blood, Bread, and Poetry

ONE OF THE CRUEL PARADOXES WE FACE TODAY IS that in this era of post-Cold War political transition, our interventions with the forces of creation—the insistent effort to improve life and to impose order on its deviations and irregularities—may well bring more harm and pain than the known devastation of violent militarism. This possibility is especially vivid when we note today's ability to isolate living genes and to transfer them from one organism to another. In a cultural milieu enthralled by technical expertise, it is not surprising that so many of those who are concerned about environmental degradation often herald advances in biotechnology, laser beams, contraceptives, or computers as *the* solution for environmental and health problems. Faith in technological progress makes us conveniently oblivious to how this technology is complicit with the forces that have produced our contemporary dilemma.

In the face of this dominant tendency that eschews values and is blind to what is lost when we insist upon being masters of nature, maintaining hope for an ecological, democratic, and egalitarian future is a constant struggle. The standard humanitarian narrative of progress brings hope to the starving, downtrodden, and ignorant masses who are miraculously uplifted by the beneficence, and above all, the technology of Western donors. Yet in my own experience, I have found it more difficult to maintain hope amidst the privileges of citizenship in a Western imperialist nation such as the United States. To be sure, the United States has Green parties and alternative grass-roots institutions that struggle to embody more egalitarian and sustainable values and practices. Nonetheless, I continually find my spirit and utopian visions dimmed here by the sight of homelessness amidst plenty, and I am painfully aware of consumerism's spread. I am often not at all sure about how to act. Here I must somehow live with the knowledge that our nation's greed and love of luxury is responsible for despoiling the Earth and wreaking havoc with cultures that are not organized around the pursuit of material abundance. My sense of the monstrous colonization practices of the U.S. and other Western nations is at times so overwhelming I am not even sure how I can support the experiments with resistance that are being so brilliantly and creatively articulated in the midst of countries who are suffering the misery and dislocation wrought by development. Indeed, upon returning from a trip to India, I found myself lapsing into a serious depression. It was only when I communicated (via computer) with a U.S. friend, also a recent returnee, who was also experiencing depression, that I was able to make the link between my depression and my quandary as to an appropriate ethic for those of us who live in the Western world.

My experiences in India taught me that many of the most interesting resistance movements are far removed from capital cities and the most prestigious institutions of higher learning and knowledge production. The critical perspectives of third world spokespersons in the new global classrooms of the West's major cities are often closer to the Eurocentric worldview that is being attacked, rather than the diverse views of their sisters and brothers who have not had such privileged access to Western education. While I have no illusions that I am capable of transcending the limitations of my own privileges, my concerns about how Eurocentric knowledge production is erasing alternative ways of knowing and doing has led me to pay particular attention to peasant women in India.

In the tumult of the Cold War's demise, the reassertion of violent nationalism had led to a certain skepticism about local small-scale solutions to the problems fostered by huge nation states and transnational corporations. I believe, however, that we must be especially attentive to alternative practices that are tied to particular place and region. Although localism offers no guarantees, the effects of the development of the global marketplace strongly suggest that egalitarian, inclusive, and ecologically sustainable practices are considerably more likely to derive from care and knowledge of local place.

Many peasant women in India, who rarely have access to the educational and class privileges of their more elite sisters, fundamentally challenge the assumptions of "first world" experts and their allies in the South. Northern experts typically promote a "politics of restructuring" that privileges greed, speed, dependency, and the power of bureaucratic expertise. In contrast, many Indian women at the grass-roots level, most especially those tribal and peasant women who still have serious ties to the land, advocate a "politics of renewal" that fosters generosity, the repair that often comes with the simple passage of time, local self-reliance, and the power of community solidarity and mutual aid. Grass-roots women of the Indian subcontinent seek to sustain and/or rebuild the diversity and security of local commons and livelihoods, challenging the project of development and enclosure of commons by the market. As the anonymous authors of *The Ecologist*'s special 1992 issue on "The Earth Summit Debacle," provocatively titled "Whose Common Future?," suggest, the developed world's market "entails an uncompromising drive toward a single global structure fitted out with mechanisms for global surveillance and global resource conversion to feed unlimited material advance."[1] Dismissing the relationships and personal values that derive from rootedness in particular places, the politics of restructuring, surely the dominant response to the contemporary ecological predicament, can only imagine a "common future" that is secured via global management and greater policing of both people and the living world.

A simple, yet profound alternative to this management and policing (which readily translates into increased policing of women's bodies) is inscribed within the exhortatory slogan of Shri Mukti Sangarsh Calwal, the Women's Liberation Movement of peasant villages in Sangli district of the state of Maharashtra: "Green Earth, Women's Power, Human Liberation." When I first heard this plea in the fall of 1991 I was thrilled. It seemed that in the United States, where identities are fractured and thinking compartmentalized, we no longer had access to such a humanistic vision. On a most grandiose level, the slogan suggests a path out of the dilemma of the Enlightenment—that technical mastery over the natural world also imprisons human capacities for polymorphous pleasures and egalitarian relationships. Shri Mukti's vision of freedom as contingent on the well-being of the Earth and the recognition of women as full persons boldly moves toward the erasure of the oppositions between human and animal, man and woman, knowledge and pleasure that have long framed Western understandings of the human condition.

Empowered by such contemporary expressions of non-Eurocentric truths, perhaps those of us in the West can more easily begin to imagine alternatives to the logic of control and mastery, alternatives that do not rush to contain and order the disorderliness of life or insist on the epistemological superiority of the transcendent, the masculine, and the visual. This recultivation of forms of knowing that have been diminished, if not eradicated, by the Enlightenment's construction of truth and the enclosure of land and peoples, creates the possibility of expanded pleasures and of mending the separation of subject and object that has produced the nightmare of a fully irradiated Earth.

It is not accidental that we find this grounded, Earth-based hope for freedom and change in a cultural and economic setting where ecological wisdom derives from the practices of daily living in rural communities. In the West, our awareness of global interconnections tends to be abstract and removed, as is so well symbolized by that cherished postmodern environmental icon, the NASA-produced whole Earth photo. For many in the United States, this high-tech image is powerfully evocative of the Earth's beauty and fragility. Yet this univocal image simultaneously conceals local knowledges and the realities of global power and domination.[2] The threats to well-being and the integrity of the biosphere produced by the imperative of growth at any cost, with its homogenizing schemes of industrialized agriculture, centralized markets, and consumer values, necessitate new images, visions, and forms of political resistance.

For the rural women of the South who worry about water, fuel, food, and fodder for sustenance, the opportunities of the global market typically represent encroachments on their livelihoods. Their fate is intimately intertwined with the well-being of the Earth, but the home these women love and struggle to protect is not the abstract whole Earth. Rather, Earth and home are the particular lands, forests and streams they personally know and care for in their daily lives. For these women the hope of liberation cannot be met with facile claims of a single earthly home; they do not fall for the myth that when we address issues of ecological devastation somehow we are all equally responsible. Nor do they imagine that there can be forms of political, cultural or economic renewal which do not account for the traditional wisdom of women.

But local as the concerns of these women are, they are also building alliances. Shri Mukti Sangarsh Calwal, for example, has worked with other peasant organizations in antidrought struggles in Sangli and adjoining districts, as well as with a larger male-led peasants' organization throughout the state—"Shetkari Sanghatana." This mass organization, led by the charismatic leader Sharad Joshi, who has a broad following across India, is primarily known for its plank of remunerative prices for peasant farmers, but in recent years Shetkari Sanghatana has also begun to agitate for natural farming, women's equal rights in property, and electing all women's panels to local governing bodies, the gram panchayat.[3] The severe droughts throughout this region linked to the practices of industrialized agriculture have led both women and men to revalue traditional agricultural practices that did not depend on the use of external inputs that needed to be bought in the marketplace. Many of these more traditional practices were typically linked to religious festivals that honor and celebrate the Earth's cycles of renewal. Shri Mukti Sangarsh, like a number of grassroots groups across India—from women fishworkers in Kerala to women tobacco workers in Nipani and tribal activists in Maharashtra—has thus begun a discussion on alternative development or counter-development from women's perspectives.[4]

Many of the activists now contend that the Green revolution in agriculture not only made the entire peasant community more dependent on dangerous pesticides, chemical fertilizers, and hybrid seeds that had to be purchased in state-controlled markets, but also deprived women of their decision-making power while increasing their labor. This degradation of traditional sustainable patterns has led some activists to call the hope of development—newly reconfigured as the hope of sustainable development—"war by other means."[5] It is argued that in traditional agriculture women maintained the seeds for planting, often deciding on where and when to plant them. In some areas they even controlled the buying and selling of cattle and sheep. Today, however, women have been displaced from the centralized economic system, and drought has increased their burden. Women's political and economic empowerment resides, not in making demands against the state, but in struggling at the local level to bring changes at the mythological, village, and household levels. Instead of insisting on access to the demeaning welfare schemes of the state, they are drawing on their collective ingenuity to restore sustainable means of survival.

The recent Laxmi Mukti campaign that has engaged activists in rural Maharashtra exemplifies the way in which contemporary ecological struggles often partake of traditional myths and symbols. This campaign for land redistribution utilizes Hindu Goddess imagery—imagery that has been for the most part scorned by urban feminists—to give visibility to its efforts. The campaign for women's land rights calls on men to put a portion of their land in the name of their wives. This struggle of liberation, "mukti," has been named Laxmi Mukti after Laxmi, the Hindu goddess of fortune. Efforts to collect information and resources in order to restore an ancient Sita temple in one of the villages that is a Shetkari Sangathana stronghold are beginning. The experimental fields where natural farming techniques that do not rely on external inputs are being investigated are termed Sita fields. The mythological goddess Sita, who, as the banished wife of the god Ram, flourished despite a painful exile, symbolizes the persisting strength of women within the confines of patriarchy. The women involved in the Laxmi Mukti campaigns are in fact revitalizing community and village forums for dealing with the issues of daily survival. In effect they are creating a way of doing democratic politics that both empowers ordinary persons and counters the managerial mentality of development experts, family planners, and the state.

The different, yet in many ways similar, struggles of women around the planet are tangible reminders that women are often the crucial leaders in maintaining communities and local ecosystems. Whereas global managers typically understand the environment in terms of what is happening in the economy, for women activists at the grass roots, the environment is what surrounds their particular homes, villages, and communities.[6] At the same time, their assorted resistances are not merely efforts to preserve the status quo, for they most typically challenge established practices and procedures that treat the Earth as a mere resource for human use. Women such as Lois Gibbs amidst the chemical toxins of Love Canal, Rachel Jones Bagby amidst the urban devastation of Philadelphia, Wangari Maathai amidst the deforested and ravaged lands of Kenya, and Medha Patkar amidst the conflicts of farmers, tribals, environmentalists, and development experts around the Narmada Dam in India, are helping to create new alliances, develop new strategies, and offer invigorating hope for diverse, sustainable communities when all hope seems to have fled.[7]

In their foregrounding of the interdependence of human and planetary well-being, the struggles of these women allow us to imagine the blossoming of new forms of adventure whose pleasure derives not from the thrill of isolated selves engaged in conquest, but from the exhilaration of engaged political participation, the play of artistic creativity, and the wonder of letting mysteries unfold. In "A Feminine Utopia," Teresa Santa Clara Gomes, deputy of the Socialist Party in the Portuguese parliament, ponders this contemporary search for new wisdom, "what remains to societies is the utopia of returning to the fundamental wisdom, the art of being amazed when confronted by the immense, unknowable, fathomless mystery that sets the rhythm of change in the universe."[8] My hope is that with this transformation of the traditional masculine taste for adventure, the thrill of sexual conquest will be replaced by the wonder of sensuous connection in all its many expressions, democratic politics will be realized, and a new, dynamic sense of peace may evolve.

Peace in its fullest sense—the ending of the global system of militarism and nation-states that are the institutionalized expression of violence, nonviolence as a maxim of daily living, and respect for the power of love and compassion—is a cornerstone of contemporary ecofeminist and Green politics. The militant, yet loving, women's encampment at the Greenham Common military installation in England, which spawned women's peace camps across the globe, still stands as one of the more important symbols of contemporary peace politics. This new politics of peace and nonviolence dos not idealize passivity. Nor does is aspire toward a static, perpetual equilibrium. Ecofeminists and Greens around the globe, from the late Petra Kelly of Germany to peace activist Corinne Kumar-D'souza of Bangalore, India, and Marxist critic and social activist Gail Omvedt of Kasegaon in rural Maharashtra, take seriously Gandhi's condemnation of passive submission to injustice. In so doing they emphasize fundamental links between ecological sanity, social justice, and the eradication of militarism, links that were not previously so well articulated by individuals and movements protesting the social injustices and Great Wars of this century.

But as the playful antics that were also part of the Greenham blockade indicate—from the belting out of songs from "The Sound of Music" at four in the morning to Irish jigs with police guards—these movements have a keen sense of adventure and play that does not partake either of Gandhi's inclination to extol suffering or his condemnation of sensuality. To quote the pagan activist Starhawk, who has reinvented the ancient spiral dance for contemporary peoples seeking to cooperatively draw on the Earth's powers,

> Gandhi was a great man, but his ideas don't always fit for a lot of us, particularly women. Gandhi said we have to accept suffering and take it in. Women have been doing that for thousands and thousands of years, and it hasn't stopped anything much—except a lot of women's lives. In some ways, it's also not ecological. Rather than absorb violence, what we need to do is to find some way to stop it and then transform it, to take the energy and turn it into creative change.[9]

Ecofeminist storytellers and activists in Kerala, India for example, have used poetry, song, pictorial representations, and street theatre to reframe Gandhian visions. Thus in the march to the southernmost point of India in 1989, where activists linked their stand against nuclear power with a stand against mechanized fishing trawlers and the demand for equitable access to clean water, women insisted that "waters must be protected if life is to be protected."[10] For these women, women's bodies are not objects for control, but sources of strength. In this emergent politics of renewal, a politics where our species' creativity holds the potential of what I like to term "re-evolution," peace and adventure are not antithetical, but mutually supportive and creative elements.

In contrast to the politics of restructuring, a politics of renewal takes little interest in control, in normalizing or containing the deviant and bizarre, for this politics understands the limits of the human mind and of rational planning on a global scale. The politics of renewal and re-evolution ask us to consider seriously the possibilities of who we might become in an unfolding universe. This politics pushes us beyond our exclusive identities (whether they be of sexuality, ethnicity, or nationality) and reminds us of our species being and our relation to cosmic forces.

Traditionally, awareness of cosmic forces has been either ignored or disdained by advocates of revolutionary change whose attention to class struggle has deafened them to notions of spirit or cosmology. Likewise, those who see possibilities in the language of evolution have neatly excised politics in a manner very similar to that of the technicians who preach restructuring. But such efforts to displace politics are fraught with peril. For one thing, problematic language of evolution can reinforce the arrogance of the canonical Darwinian view that posits human beings as the highest expression of creation.[11] Our evolution into more loving, reflective, and ecologically conscious beings, which

New Agers long for, is a worthy vision, but its realization is by no means inevitable. We cannot rely on the playing out of some higher natural law. Humans, most especially white ones of the North, must consciously decide to reimagine ourselves. The scope of personal and institutional change that is necessary cannot be contained either within traditional notions of revolutionary change that emphasize the seizure of state power, or the technical plans of contemporary advocates of restructuring who prefer the reform of state power to facilitate global markets. Given our patterns of overconsumption, living lightly on the planet will necessarily mean doing with less materially. At the level of our personal and community lives, such a transformation could well be experienced as joyful and spiritually liberating. Less does not have to be understood as deprivation. As Jane Bennett puts it in her argument for a "fractious holism," which tolerates otherness in nature and the social order, "What justification can an ethic that seeks to express a fractious world give for its desire to tread lightly? . . . We should tread lightly because it is the wisest orientation to a world upon which we depend but which we cannot fully comprehend or control. . . . Human existence upon the planet is precarious, not guaranteed."[12] The challenge is to repair and create democratic, self-reliant, frugal, and egalitarian institutions that primarily trade through more barterized and face to face modes of exchange, rather than the exclusively monetized and abstract modes of exchange we have come to understand as trade. Such institutions would be capable of surviving without the known securities of the current nation-state system. Of course this is not a simple task, but such shifts are already occurring in local places across the globe. Across the globe, we can find the re-invention of community-based networks for the cooperative care of children, public safety, gardens, spiritual needs, and burial preparation, to the different efforts to transform travel and adventure through practices of responsible tourism, the invention of bioregional economic networks that utilize their own currencies, and the maintenance or creation of local craft markets where information, services and self-produced goods are exchanged.[13] And to those who would raise the spectre or anarchy (a false understanding of what anarchists working in the collectivist tradition intended), I would take note of Thomas Kuehl's provocative suggestion that "neither nature nor humanity is predisposed to the workings of the state. . . . Where the majority of sovereignty theorists present humans and nature as objects readily available for the imposition of sovereignty, a Foucauldian analysis draws out the work that must be done to both in the name of sovereignty."[14]

The process of re-evolution is synergistic, more like the ripples of unfolding spirals or seashells, than the additive or linear processes we typically associate with evolutionary notions of change. We must forge new metaphors like Starhawk's spiral dance to generate visions of horizontal linkages and unpredictability. In dance, integral to the rituals of almost all indigenous cultures, the rhythmic changes and energies of our bodies are linked to the Earth's cycles of renewal. In expanding and enriching our sensory capacities, the politics of re-evolution may well strengthen our bonds to the Earth and each other, allowing us to experience in positive ways what the West names as the otherness of nature.

Within this emergent politics, the traditional polarities of modern politics are reframed. I have suggested in this chapter, ecofeminists, Greens, and bioregionalists are often sympathetic to traditional practices and ways of living. Vernacular knowledge is highly respected and valued. Unlike Enlightenment modernizers who focus on the hope of the future by denigrating the past, the politics of renewal and re-evolution create new visions by drawing on the wisdom of tradition.

Here again there is an important kinship with Gandhi. As the contemporary activist and editor of *Manushi* women's magazine, Madhu Kishwar, notes, according to Gandhi, "It is good to swim in the waters of tradition, but to sink in them is suicide."[15] Tradition must be drawn upon as a guide, but we must not let it limit our thinking as we respond to new conditions. For grass-roots activists in India confronting contemporary energy needs, the tradition of making use of the Earth's riches may mean the invention of compost-to-energy-converter technologies that use the animal dung and discarded vegetation which development has defined as waste. Indeed for many activists in the appropriate-technology movement, locally produced biomass is central to the vision of village-centered societies.

Within the politics of renewal, an awareness of the people and practices that preceded us is necessary to determine the repercussions of our present activities and technologies. By resisting our modern language of control, and by invoking respect for the fertility of the soil, our bodies, and the communities that nourish our hearts and minds, ecofeminists and Greens seek to sustain both the living Earth and all her unique creatures. Nor is this commitment to diversity an abstract ideal or some easy substitute for eternal truth. Diversity is basic to ecosystemic well-being. By opposing the homogenizing, elitist vision of technological control with a more complex understanding of diversity and the practices of indigenous peoples who honor the continuity and sacredness of life, ecofeminists and Greens struggle to preserve yet transform community and democracy in the modern world.

Rather than bemoan the end of nature, we humans, women and men, need to re-evolve into beings who prefer our local gardens. We must resist the call of Western tradition to bring enlightenment to all the planet. Paradoxical though it may seem, a respect for fertility—in all its diverse vegetative, social, and imaginative forms—may be the most prudent, moral, and politically effective means for surviving into the twenty-first century. The sorry history of the language of control tells us that the difficult, yet essential, task of creating communities that honor the manifold wonders of fertility is the primary task before us. The living Earth beckons.

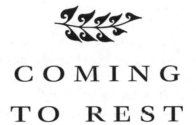

COMING
TO REST

The entire world is a very narrow bridge. The essential thing is to have no fear at all.

ATTRIBUTED TO NAHMAN OF BRATZLAV

The great essence will flower in our lives
and expand throughout the world.
May we learn to let it shine through so we can augment its glory.
We praise, we continue to praise, and yet, whatever it is we praise,
is quite beyond the grasp of all these words
and symbols that point us towards it.
We know, and yet we do not know,
May great peace pour forth from heavens for us, for all Israel,
for all who struggle toward truth.
May that which makes harmony in the cosmos above,
bring peace within and between us, and to all who dwell on this earth,
and let us say, Amen.

RABBI BURT JACOBSON,
"Kaddish, Mourner's Prayer," from the Aquarian Minyan Siddur

We are different from one another
Woman is different from Man.
Humans and animals are different too
All in Nature's wondrous plan.
Day and night, darkness and light,
The rays of moon and sun,

We call holy all of these
A blessing is each and every one.

Baruh beruhah, kadosh kedoshah
Our voices are different
some quiet, some strong.
Our voices are lovely
Some old and some young.

We call holy all of these
A blessing is each and every one.

LEILA GAL BERNER,
"Hevdelim," from "Song and Grace after Meals"

THIS BOOK WAS BEING FINISHED AS THE GREAT FLOODS of 1993 tore through cemeteries that had been built on the flood plains of the Mississippi, sending safely secured burial coffins, many of which likely had guarantees to be airtight and watertight for fifty years or more, floating downstream. I became aware of some of the peculiarities of non-native North American burial practices during this flood which had no precedent within the memory of modern dam-makers, because I was confronting my own mother's physical degeneration and impending death as the torrential rains fell.

The concerns that animated this book were born out of my queries regarding Western feminist rhetoric about controlling our bodies. This expression of women's freedom, though forged out of the necessary struggle to resist men's power over women, nonetheless still partakes of our larger culture's denial of the cycles of birth, death, and renewal. My questioning pushed me to recast contemporary feminism from an ecological perspective that seemed to adequately acknowledge the wisdom and virtue of "living within limits."[1] Yet as I delved further I found that much of the modern environmental movement sought to save nature while relying on a language that had no respect for women, nature's own agency, or the voices of the socially disempowered.

My initial concerns were the dilemmas the language of control posed for practices of birth prevention and the cultural politics of women's identity construction. Though we lived in the age of the sexuated body and ever more efficient modes of birth control, I worried about the loss of our ability to love, and to experience the pleasures of community-building and communion with the world around. Gradually I came to realize that these problems were even more complicated than I had first imagined, for, as we've seen, how we understand our own bodies is intimately related to how we seek to manage and organize the Earth's bounty. In neither case do we acknowledge the cycles of living and dying. Throughout the course of writing this book, I became keenly aware of the necessity of new languages, practices, and rituals to counter the invasive surgeries, therapies, and toxic pharmaceuticals of Western medicine.

Yet it wasn't until my aging and frail mother lapsed into a coma after a massive stroke that I began to sense how profoundly I still negotiated the world through a reliance on reason that was divorced from bodily cycles. Now I had to face the fact that the narrative I had constructed for my mother's life—that her body would remain alive until she was very old—was not the one the creator intended. My mother's younger sister told me that she too had had imagined that her oldest sister would live to be a hundred, outliving the three remaining sisters of the original group of six. In realizing that something else was intended, the notion of a creator reentered my vocabulary.

In the final weeks of my mother's life, I suddenly found myself dealing with how our culture's technologies of control had sought to reorganize fertility but also death. Where just a few years earlier I had been resisting the technologies that sought to introduce "quality control" to birthing and birth, now I found myself resisting their application to dying and death. And when I saw with my own eyes how my mother fought to remove the tubes of life modern medicine had produced, I knew that in her unconscious state she was resisting as well. Yet because my own knowledge of death was so shaped by the images I had seen in movies and television, I was puzzled and frightened when she lived peacefully without food or water for eight days.

When the phone rang at one in the morning, I realized that my mother had chosen to die at the opening of the tenth day as the calendar marked the Sabbath. I ran down to hold her hand one last time. When I witnessed the peace that had returned to her face after the belabored breathing and death sounds of just a few hours earlier, I suddenly saw in the pulsations of her enlarged Adam's apple a mirror of the pushing and throbbing of the birth process (when it is allowed). I who, despite my ten-year engagement with ecological learning, rarely invoked the language of blessing felt I had somehow been blessed by this opportunity to observe a nexus point of life and death. Abraham Heschel's view of Shabbat came to mind:

> To set apart one day a week for freedom, a day on which we would not use the instruments which have been so easily turned into weapons of destruction, a day of being with ourselves, a day of detachment from the vulgar, of independence of external obligation, a day on which we stop worshipping the idols of technical civilization, a day on which we use no money, a day of armistice in the economic struggle with our fellow men and the forces of nature—is there any institution that holds out a greater hope for man's progress than the Sabbath? The solution of mankind's most vexing problem will not be found in renouncing technical civilization, but in attaining some degree of independence from it.[2]

Returning home after my mother's difficult passage, I found myself deriving comfort from my reading of the Jewish traditions' burial rituals. I had always known that Jewish law dictated that the dead be buried as soon as possible; in my reading I learned that "Jewish burial practice, since the fourth century C.E. rabbinic reforms, places emphasis on speed, simplicity, and an explicit confrontation with the facts of finitude."[3] But I had never quite realized how ecological Jewish practices were. Jews had adapted to dominant North American customs with our prescription that the coffin be made of wood so as to enable to corpse to return and nourish the soil as quickly as possible. A friend reported that in Israel Jews simply wrap a corpse in a shroud, then place it on twigs and allow it to slip into the ground. The ancient Jewish concepts of "tumah," "the result of our confrontation with the fact of our own mortality," and "taharah," "the result of our reaffirmation of our own immortality," were vivid reminders that "all things die and are reborn continually." I learned that one of the ways of making contact with tumah was through touching the inanimate shell of a human corpse. Tumah was not pollution, thus a corpse was not to be treated with dread and avoidance; indeed the care of the dead is a special mitzvah or holy deed.[4] I was overwhelmed when I learned that my local community had enough members who knew of the power of this mitzvah that they had been able to recreate a traditional, totally nonprofit Hevra Kadisha (Holy Brotherhood) that was responsible for preparing the dead for burial.

With the reports of flooding in the Midwest a constant backdrop to my immersion in the Jewish rituals of death and dying, I recalled that when I first learned that many traditions had stories of great floods comparable to the story of Noah, I believed that if the tales of my people were not unique then that was certain proof that there was no creator.

Today I am more inclined to see the immense wisdom that is embedded in many different spiritual traditions, and I see the Noah story as a warning of what can happen when humans exercise imprudent and reckless dominion over the Earth. At the same time, I worry that the very occurrence of the great flood of 1993 may be used by environmentalists to fuel the apocalyptic, endtime mode of thinking of the modern environmental movement that is mostly antithetical to the project of creating a more democratic, socially just, and ecologically sustainable world. In my view the occurrence of a flood of biblical proportions in our contemporary technical civilization is both a pointed reminder of the limits of our control, and an indication that beginnings and ends are intimately related to each other. My sense is that disasters and repair and mending have always been part of the story of the world, and it is our task to continue to be repairers, however undramatic and unnewsworthy such practices might be.

One of the arguments of this book has been that ecofeminist politics learns from the wisdom of traditional practices. The occasion of my mother's passing enabled me to reflect upon the ecological teachings embedded within the tradition within which I have been brought up and which I had in many ways resisted much of my adult life. After studying the intelligence of age-old customs in India and of indigenous peoples around the globe, my intellectual knowledge of Jewish traditions became embodied in my daily experience of the world only very recently.

Of course there are many strands of thought that constitute Judaism, and these have changed through the ages. Returning to my roots in this postmodern era I am particularly drawn to interpretations offered by sages and artists who honor mystery and worry about the remaking of relationships between women and men. Thus Arthur Waskow's interpretation of the significance of feminism for the Jewish observance of Shabbat is particularly compelling:

> Under the new conditions of new forms of relationship
> between women and men, the full celebration of shabbat
> may require that, on that day, there be an even fuller sharing
> of nurturance and community, an even more conscious shat-
> tering of separate roles of women and men, than on the six
> workdays . . . if shabbat entered the conscious practice of

the people of Israel as a first step in reversing the post-Edenic curse upon Adam that he must toil in the sweat of his brow to wrest bread from the hostile earth, then it may also become a first step in reversing the post-Edenic curse upon Eve: that she must be ruled over by her husband and must suffer childbearing and painful labor.[5]

In our era, which is struggling to come to terms both with the challenges of feminism and the dangers of technological triumph, Judaism, and religion more generally, have been reinvigorated by the recasting of traditional tales, the borrowing of tales across traditions, and the effort to make these tales more fitting to the challenges we face. As an ecofeminist, I believe the most profound challenge we face is how to name wrongdoing without destroying the wrongdoer, how to live as equals with other peoples and the Earth while acknowledging our differences and diversity. In the practical cosmology of ecofeminism, mystery and diversity are the occasion for celebration—a source for our freedom and our hope for the future.

N O T E S

CHAPTER I
Feminism, Fertility, and the Living Earth

1. See Laura Lederer, ed., *Take Back the Night: Women and Pornography* (New York: William Morrow and Co., 1980).
2. Susan Griffin, *Pornography and Silence: Culture's Revenge against Nature* (New York: Harper and Row, 1981).
3. Susan Griffin, *Made from this Earth* (London: Women's Press, 1981).
4. See Cynthia Hamilton, "Women, Home, and Community: The Struggle in an Urban Environment," in *Reweaving the World: The Emergence of Ecofeminism*, ed. Irene Diamond and Gloria Feman Orenstein (San Francisco: Sierra Club, 1990), pp. 215–22.
5. See Werner Hulsberg, *The German Greens: A Social and Political Profile,* trans. Gus Fagan (London: Verso, 1988). Charlene Spretnak and Fritjof Capra, *Green Politics: The Global Promise* (Santa Fe: Bear and Co., 1984).
6. Lewis Hyde, in *The Gift: Imagination and the Erotic Life of Property* (New York: Random House, 1983), writes, "When we see that we are actors in natural cycles, we understand that what nature gives to us is influenced by what we give to nature. . . . The forest's abundance is in fact a consequence of man's treating its wealth as a gift" (p. 19).
7. Carol P. Christ, *Laughter of Aphrodite: Reflections on a Journey to the Goddess* (San Francisco: Harper and Row, 1987), p. 219.
8. "Our Bodies, Ourselves" is the title of a popular handbook on

women's health by the Boston Women's Health Collective which has been translated into many languages and is used by grass-roots feminist health clinics around the world. "Woman's Body, Woman's Right" is the title of the definitive feminist history of birth control in America by Linda Gordon. "Sexuality is to feminism" is from Catharine MacKinnon's "Feminism, Marxism, Method, and the State: An Agenda for Theory," *Signs* 7 (Spring 1982).

9. See Nancy Hartsock, *Money, Sex and Power: Toward a Feminist Historical Materialism* (New York: Longman, 1983); Dorothy Smith, *The Every Day World as Problematic* (Boston: Northeastern University Press, 1987); Mary O'Brien, *The Politics of Reproduction* (Boston: Routledge and Kegan Paul, 1981); Charlotte Perkins Gilman, *Women and Economics* (Boston-Small Maynard & Co., 1898).

10. Rosalind Petchesky, *Abortion and Woman's Choice: The State, Sexuality, and Reproductive Freedom* (New York: Longman, 1984), p. 3.

11. Linda Singer, *Erotic Welfare: Sexual Theory and Politics in the Age of Epidemic* (New York: Routledge, 1993), p. 36.

12. For an important exception, see Germaine Greer, *Sex and Destiny: The Politics of Human Fertility* (New York: Harper and Row, 1984).

13. Thomas Malthus, *An Essay on the Principle of Population* (New York: Norton, 1976).

CHAPTER 2
Bodies, Sex, and Feminist Politics

1. For material on overreliance on our visual sense, see Evelyn Fox Keller and Christine R. Grontkowski, "The Mind's Eye," in *Discovering Reality: Feminist Perspectives on Epistemology, Metaphysics, Methodology, and Philosophy of Science*, ed. Sandra Harding and Merrill B. Hintikka (Dordrecht, Holland: D. Reidel, 1983), pp. 207–24; Carolyn Merchant, *Ecological Revolutions: Nature, Gender, and Science in New England* (Chapel Hill: University of North Carolina Press, 1989), and Lorraine Code, *What Can She Know?* (Ithaca: Cornell University Press, 1991).

2. Simone de Beauvoir, *The Second Sex*, trans. and ed. H. M. Parshley (New York: Knopf, 1952).

3. Juliet Mitchell, *Woman's Estate* (New York: Pantheon Books, 1971), p. 35.

4. Jane Bennett, *Unthinking Faith and Enlightenment: Nature and the State in a Post-Hegelian Era* (New York: New York University Press, 1987), p. 147.

5. For a discussion of how some feminists have opposed waiting periods designed to protect poor women, see Linda Gordon, *Woman's Body, Woman's Right,* 2d ed. (New York: Penguin, 1990).

6. Az Carmen, "Why Historical Anger Is Good," unpublished paper, University of Oregon, 1993, in possession of author. Native women's experiences of sterilization have yet to be fully documented. See U.S. General Accounting Office Report to Hon. James G. Abourezk, B164031, November 1976; Janet Larson, "And Then There Were None: IHS Sterilization Practices," *Christian Century* 94 (1977), pp. 61–63; Brint Dillingham, "Indian Women and IHS Sterilization Practices," *American Indian Journal* 3, 1 (January 1977), pp. 27–28; for overviews of involuntary sterilization more generally in the U.S., see Philip P. Reilly, *The Surgical Solution: A History of Involuntary Sterilization in the United States* (Baltimore: Johns Hopkins University Press, 1991); Committee for Abortion Rights and Against Sterilization Abuse, *Women Under Attack: Victories, Backlash, and the Fight for Reproductive Rights,* ed. Susan E. Davis (Boston: South End Press, 1988); Thomas M. Shapiro, *Population Control Policies: Women, Sterilization, and Reproductive Choice* (Philadelphia: Temple University Press, 1985); for international sterilization abuse, see Betsy Hartmann, *Reproductive Rights and Wrongs: The Global Politics of Population Control and Contraceptive Choice* (New York: Harper and Row, 1987); for a particularly compelling account of abuses in India see the film *Something Like a War,* by Deepa Dhanraj, D&N Productions, Bangalore 560001.

7. For the coercive use of Norplant in the United States, see Chapter 3. See also "Poverty and Norplant: Can Contraception Reduce the Underclass?", *Philadelphia Inquirer,* Sept. 13, 1991, and Julia R. Scott, "Norplant: Its Impact on Poor Women and Women of Color," Public Policy/Education Office, National Black Women's Health Project. "Native Americans Uncover Norplant and Sterilization Abuses," *Ms. Magazine* (September/October 1993), p. 27; Alta Chara, "Medicine and the Law: Mandatory Contraception," *The Lancet* 339 (May 1992), pp. 1104–5. The state of New Jersey has also passed Welfare 'reform' legislation which denies benefits to children born to women already receiving public assistance.

8. See Mayra Buvinic, Margaret A. Lycette, and William Paul McGreevey, eds., *Women and Poverty in the Third World* (Baltimore (Johns Hopkins University Press, 1983); Barbara C. Gelpi, ed., *Women and Poverty* (Chicago: University of Chicago Press, 1986); Diane Schaffer, "The Feminization of Poverty: Prospects for an International Feminist Agenda," in Ellen Boneparth and Emily Stoper, eds., *Women, Power, and Public Policy* (New York: Pergamon, 1988); Jeanne Vickers, *Women and the World Economic Crises* (London: Zed Books, 1991)); and Paul E. Zopf, Jr., *American Women in Poverty* (New York: Greenwood Press, 1989).

9. Adrienne Rich, *Of Woman Born: Motherhood as Experience and Institution* (New York: Norton, 1976).

10. Nancy C. M. Hartsock, *Money, Sex and Power: Toward a Feminist Historical Materialism* (New York: Longman, 1983); Maria Mies, *Patriarchy and Accumulation on a World Scale: Women in the International Division of Labor* (London: Atlantic Highlands, 1986); Sara Ruddick, *Maternal Thinking: Toward a Politics of Peace* (Boston: Beacon Press, 1989); and Julia Kristeva, "Women's Time," *Signs* 7, no. 1 (Autumn 1981).

11. Hartsock, *Money, Sex and Power*, p. 247.

12. Ruddick, *Maternal Thinking*, p. 195.

13. As stated by the chorus in Euripides, *The Bacchae*, trans. Michael Cacoyannis (New York: New American Library, 1982).

14. Michel Foucault, *The History of Sexuality*, vol. 1, trans. Robert Hurley (New York: Pantheon, 1978), p. 78.

15. Catharine MacKinnon, "Sexual Pornography and Method: Pleasure Under Patriarchy," *Ethics* 99 (January 1989); Andrea Dworkin, *Pornography: Men Possessing Women* (New York: Perigee, 1981); Andrea Dworkin and Catharine MacKinnon, *Pornography and Civil Rights: A New Day for Women's Equality* (Minneapolis: Organizing Against Pornography, 1988); Carol Vance, "More Danger, More Pleasure: A Decade after the Barnard Sexuality Conference," in Carole Vance, ed., *Pleasure and Danger: Exploring Female Sexuality*, 2d ed. (London: Pandora Press, 1992); Kate Roiphe, *The Morning After: Sex, Fear, and Feminism on Campus* (Boston: Little Brown, 1993); Ellen Willis, *No More Nice Girls: Counter Cultural Essays* (Hanover: Wesleyan University Press, 1992).

16. It is interesting to note here that while Foucault is very critical of the way in which human sciences have operated, his polemics have not been directed at physical sciences. In contrast,

feminist criticism has interrogated the way in which gender hierarchy was encoded within the construction of modern science. See, for example, Evelyn Fox Keller, *Reflections on Gender and Science* (New Haven: Yale University Press, 1985); Vandana Shiva, *Staying Alive* (New Delhi: Kali for Women, 1988); and Susan Griffin, *Woman and Nature: The Roaring Inside Her* (San Francisco: Harper and Row, 1978). For a discussion of how as modern science developed in the West the understanding of the earth as a living organism changed to that of a dead machine, see Carolyn Merchant, *The Death of Nature: Women, Ecology and the Scientific Revolution* (New York: Harper and Row, 1980).

17. Foucault, *History of Sexuality,* p. 107.

18. Ibid., p. 136.

19. Ibid., p. 155.

20. Bernard Weinraub, "Women's Roles in Films Draw Women's Fire," *The New York Times,* June 2, 1993, p. B1.

21. Germaine Greer, *Sex and Destiny: The Politics of Human Fertility* (New York: Harper and Row, 1984), p. 235.

22. For material on ecofeminism, see Judith Plant, "Searching for Common Ground: Ecofeminism and Bioregionalism,: in *Reviewing the World: the Emergence of Ecofeminism,* ed. Irene Diamond and Gloria Feman Orenstein (San Francisco: Sierra Club, 1990), and Leonie Caldecott and Stephanie Leland, eds., *Reclaim the Earth: Women Speak Out for Life on Earth* (London: The Women's Press, 1983) and *The Ecologist* 22, no. 1 (January/February 1992).

23. See Carol Gilligan, *In a Different Voice: Psychological Theory and Women's Development* (Cambridge, Mass.: Harvard University Press, 1982), pp. 42–43.

24. Catharine MacKinnon, *The Sexual Harassment of Women* (New Haven: Yale University Press, 1987); Charlene Spretnak, ed., *The Politics of Women's Spirituality* (New York: Doubleday, 1982); Susan Brownmiller, *Against Our Will: Men, Women, and Rape* (New York: Simon and Schuster, 1975); *The Laughter of Aphrodite: Reflections on a Journey to the Goddess* (San Francisco: Harper and Row, 1987).

25. Shulamith Firestone, *Dialectic of Sex: The Case for Feminist Revolution* (New York: Bantam Books, 1971).

26. Adrienne Rich, *Of Woman Born* (New York: Bantam Books, 1976); Mary Daly, *Gyn/Ecology, the Metaethics of Radical Feminism* (Boston: Beacon Press, 1978); Susan Griffin, *Woman and Nature: The Roaring Inside Her* (New York: Harper

and Row, 1978); Audre Lorde, *Sister Outsider: Essays and Speeches* (Trumansburg, N.Y.: Crossing Press, 1984); Alice Walker, *In Search of Our Mother's Gardens* (San Diego: Harcourt Brace Jovanovich, 1983); Starhawk, *Dreaming the Dark: Magic, Sex and Politics* (Boston: Beacon Press, 1982); Paula Gunn Allen, *The Sacred Hoop: Recovering the Feminine In American Indian Traditions* (Boston: Beacon Press, 1986).

27. Susan Griffin, *Woman of Power 1,* 1 (Spring 1984), p. 35.

28. For material on women's peace movements, see Adrienne Harris and Ynestra King, eds. *Rocking the Ship of State: Toward a Feminist Peace Politics* (Boulder: Westview, 1989); Lynne Jones, ed., *Keeping the Peace* (London: Women's Press, 1983); Petra Kelly, *Fighting for Hope* (Boston: South End Press, 1984), and Anne Seller, "Greenham: A Concrete Reality," *Frontiers* 8 (1985), pp. 26–31.

29. See, for example, Christ, *Laughter of Aphrodite;* Charlene Spretnak, *The Politics of Women's Spirituality: Essays on the Rise of Spiritual Power within the Feminist Movement* (Garden City, N.Y.: Doubleday, 1981); Marija Gimbutas, *The Goddesses and Gods of Old Europe, 6500–3500 B.C.: Myths, Legends, and Cult Images* (Berkeley: University of California Press, 1982).

30. Carolyn Merchant, *Ecological Revolutions: Nature, Gender, and Science in New England* (Chapel Hill: University of North Carolina Press, 1989), p. 58.

31. Gayatri Spivak, in *Other Words: Essays in Cultural Politics* (New York: Methuen, 1987), uses the phrase "irresponsible dreamers."

32. Donna Haraway, "A Manifesto for Cyborgs: Science, Technology, and Socialist Feminism in the 1980s," *Socialist Review* 80 (1985), pp. 65–107.

33. Lorraine Code, *What Can She Know? Feminist Theory and the Construction of Knowledge* (Ithaca: Cornell University Press, 1991).

34. Drucilla Cornell, *Beyond Accommodation* (New York: Routledge, 1991), pp. 168–69.

35. See Carol Van Strum, *Bitter Fog: Herbicides and Human Rights* (San Francisco: Sierra Club, 1983); Lois Gibbs, *Love Canal: My Story* (Albany: SUNY Press, 1982); David Weir, *The Bhopal Syndrome: Pesticides, Environment and Health* (San Francisco: Sierra Club, 1987); Rachel L. Bagby, "Daughters of Growing Things," in Diamond and Orenstein, eds., *Reweaving the World.*

36. For discussion of the relationship between the Chipko and the Bishnoi women, see Vandana Shiva, *Staying Alive: Women, Ecology, and Development* (New Delhi: Kali for Women, 1988).
37. For more on maldevelopment, see Vandana Shiva, *Staying Alive*. For more on antidevelopment, see Maria Mies, "Women and Development: Conceptual Issues from a Global Perspective," paper presented at the Consultative Workshop: Women, Development and Mountain Resources, Kathmandu, November 1989. For more on counter-development, see Helena Norbert-Hodge, *Ancient Futures: Learning from Ladakh* (San Francisco: Sierra Club, 1991). See also Gabriele Dietrich, *Women's Movement in India* (Bangalore: Breakthrough Publications, 1988), and *Reflections on the Women's Movement in India: Religion, Ecology and Development* (New Delhi: Horizon Books, 1992); Bina Agarwal, "The Gender and Environment Debate: Lessons from India," *Feminist Studies* 18, no. 1 (Spring 1992), pp. 119–58, and Gail Omvedt, *Reinventing Revolution: New Social Movements and the Socialist Tradition in India* (Armonk, N.Y.: M.E. Sharpe, 1993).
38. Andrew Ross, "The Ecology of Images," *The South Atlantic Quarterly* 91, no. 1 (Winter 1992).
39. For critiques of Green consumerism from an ecofeminist perspective, see H. Patricia Hynes, "The Race to Save the Planet, Will Women Lose," *Women's Studies International Forum* 12, no. 5 (1991), pp. 473–78, and Catriona Sandilands, "On 'Green' Consumerism: Environmental Privatization and 'Family Values',", *Canadian Women's Studies* (Spring 1993), 13, no. 3, pp. 45–47.
40. We can note here such ingenious bureaucratic incentive systems as in Rajistan, India, where family planning providers are offered "free air travel for Global Tour for 7 days" if they exceed their annual targets for sterilization. *Development for Whom? A Critique of Women's Development Programmes* (New Delhi: Saheli, October 1991). Christa Wichterich points out that "under conditions of poverty where the premium (for sterilization) is greater than the monthly wage of an agricultural worker, it is pointless to describe the women's' decisions as voluntary." Christa Wichterich, "From the Struggle Against 'Overpopulation' to the Industrialization of Human Production," in *Issues in Reproductive and Genetic Engineering* 1, no. 1 (1988), pp. 21–30. See also Charanjit Ahuja, "To Meet Family Planning Targets, Tubectomy Forced on 61-year-old Widow," *Indian Express* (Jan. 25, 1992); Farida Akhter, *Depopulating Bangladesh*

(Dhaka, Bangladesh: Ubinig, 1989); Betsy Hartmann, *Reproductive Rights and Wrongs: The Global Politics of Population Control and Contraceptive Choice* (New York: Harper and Row, 1987); and Angana Parekh, "How Sterile the Sterilisation Programme . . .," *Indian Express* (Feb. 14, 1992).
41. Wichterich, "From The Struggle Against 'Overpopulation' to the Industrialization of Human Production."
42. Hannah Arendt, *The Human Condition* (Chicago: University of Chicago Press, 1958), p. 2.

CHAPTER 3
Sex without Consequences

1. In "The Elimination of Medieval Birth Control and the Witch Trials of Modern Times." *International Journal of Women's Studies 5*, no. 3, pp. 193–214, Gunnar Heinsohn and Otto Steiger contend that "the witch massacres are attributable to the political determination to eradicate the medieval knowledge of birth control in order to force women to conceive." For premodern practices, see John H. Riddle, *Contraception and Abortion from the Ancient World to the Renaissance* (Cambridge: Harvard University Press, 1992).
2. Linda Gordon, *Woman's Body, Woman's Right: Birth Control in America* (New York: Pantheon, 1978); Rosalind Petchesky, *Abortion and Women's Choice* (Boston: Longman, 1984).
3. See Gordon, *Woman's Body,* chap. 5, for a discussion of voluntary motherhood.
4. William Leach, *True Love and Perfect Union* (New York: Basic Books, 1980), p. 43.
5. Lucinda Chandler, "Marital Equality," in *Revolution,* July 20, 1871, as quoted in Leach, *True Love and Perfect Union,* p. 89.
6. Ibid., p. 89,
7. Ibid.
8. For a fuller discussion of Sheppard-Towner, see Rothman, *Woman's Proper Place: A History of Changing Ideals and Practices, 1870 to the Present* (New York: Basic Books, 1978); J. Stanley Lemons, *The Women Citizen: Social Feminism in the 1920's* (Urbana: University of Illinois Press, 1973), chap. 6.
9. Rothman, *Woman's Proper Place,* pp. 200–209.
10. Mary Ryan, *Motherhood in America,* 2d ed. (Philadelphia: Franklin and Watts, 1978), chap. 5.

11. Rothman, *Woman's Proper Place,* chap. 5, describes the shifts in popular advice manuals of the 1920s.
12. Ibid., p. 191.
13. Ibid., pp. 200–209.
14. For a more general discussion of the consolidation of the medical profession's power, see Paul Starr, *The Social Transformation of American Medicine* (New York: Basic Books, 1982), chap. 3; for a fuller discussion of how political conservatism contributed to the defeat of Sheppard-Towner, see Rothman, *Woman's Proper Place,* pp. 142–51; Lemons, *The Woman Citizen,* pp. 171–76; and Richard W. and Dorothy C. Wertz, *Lying In: A History of Childbirth in America* (New York: Schocken, 1977), pp. 206–210.
15. John Horgan, "Eugenics Revisited," in *Scientific American* (June 1993), p. 130.
16. Ruth Hubbard and Elijah Wald, *Exploding the Gene Myth: How Genetic Information is Produced and Manipulated by Scientists, Physicians, Employers, Insurance Companies, Educators, and Law Enforcers* (Boston: Beacon Press, 1993), p. 21.
17. Sanger, as quoted in Gordon, *Woman's Body,* p. 287.
18. Gordon, *Woman's Body,* p. 345.
19. See Gordon, *Woman's Body,* chap. 10, and Petchesky, *Abortion and Woman's Choice,* p. 208.
20. This survey is discussed in Charles Westoff, "The Fertility of the American Population," in Ronald Friedman, ed., *Population: The Vital Revolution* (Garden City: Doubleday, 1964), pp. 110–12.
21. Bonnie Mass, *Population Target: The Political Economy of Population Control in Latin America* (Toronto: Women's Press, 1976).
22. For material on overzealous family planning recruiters in China, see John S. Aird, *Slaughter of the Innocents* (Washington, D.C.: The AEI Press, 1990). See also Betsy Hartmann, *Reproductive Rights and Wrongs: The Global Politics of Population Control and Reproductive Choice* (New York: Harper and Row, 1987), for a more general overview.
23. As quoted in Greer, *Sex and Destiny,* p. 437.
24. Anne L. Harper, "Teenage Sexuality and Public Policy: An Agenda for Gender Education," in Irene Diamond, ed., *Families, Politics and Public Policy: A Feminist Dialogue on Women and the State* (New York: Longman, 1983), p. 221.
25. The Carter Administration assembled a large interagency team to come up with appropriate policy recommendations. In

August of 1977 that team responded with a set of recommendations that reflected the prevailing paradigm in the family planning
community: more family planning prevention services and the
reduction of barriers to services. The specific recommendations of
more abortion counseling and referral services and more encour-
agement to the states to permit adolescents to receive contraceptive services without parental consent did not appeal to either
Carter or his Catholic Secretary of Health and Human Services,
Joseph P. Califano. Instead, the Secretary returned to a policy
option that an earlier HEW Special Task Force had suggested.
This group had recommended a Family Development Program
that would "provide practical, ethical, and politically viable alternatives to abortion" and would result in "verifiable improvements in family life." The suggested program of comprehensive
service centers for pregnant teenagers drew on one that had begun
at the Johns Hopkins Medical School for adolescent obstetrical
patients. The Hopkins program provided support services not
normally available to pregnant adolescents: prenatal educational
and medical services coupled with educational and vocational
counseling and postnatal services for both adolescent mothers and
infants. See Gilbert Steiner, *The Futility of Family Policy* (Washington, D.C.: Brookings Institute, 1981).
26. Maris Vinovskis, in *An "Epidemic" of Adolescent Pregnancy* (New York: Oxford University Press, 1988), estimated that
there were 120,000 responses, of which I read approximately
750.
27. Michel Foucault, *Foucault Live (Interviews, 1966–84)* (New
York: Semiotext(e), 1989), p. 145.
28. For a critique of the language of reproductive rights from a
feminist and Marxist third world perspective, see Farida Akhter,
"The Eugenic and Racist Premise of Reproductive Rights and
Population Control," in *Issues in Reproductive and Genetic Engineering: Journal of International Feminist Analysis* 5, no. 1
(1992), pp. 1–8.
29. R. J. Apfel and S. M. Fischer, *DES and the Dilemmas of
Modern Medicine* (New Haven: Yale University Press, 1984); A.
L. Herbst and H. A. Berne, *Developmental Effects of Diethylstilbestrol (DES) in Pregnancy* (New York: Thieme Stratton,
1981). Theo Colburn, Frederick S. vom Saal, and Ana M. Soto, in
a major report, "Developmental Effects of Endocrine-Disrupting
Chemicals in Wildlife and Humans," *Environmental Health Perspectives* 101, no. 5 (October 1993), argue that DES-exposed

humans "serve as a model for exposure during early life to any estrogenic chemical, including pollutants in the environment that are estrogen agonists." Their concern is that numerous types of these chemicals have been released into the environment since World War II and that "endocrine-disrupting effects are not currently considered in assessing risks to humans, domestic animals, and wildlife." The emphasis in the report is that the effects of such chemicals are often long-term or transgenerational.

30. For a discussion of these methods as they relate to gender relations, see Robert A. Jonas, "Birth Control in a Culture of Changing Sex Roles: The NFP Experience," doctoral dissertation, Harvard Graduate School of Education, 1983; Kristin Luker, *Abortion and the politics of Motherhood* (Berkeley: University of California Press, 1984), pp. 211–12; Susan Bell et al., "Reclaiming Reproductive Control: A Feminist Approach to Fertility Consciousness," *Science for the People* 12, no. 1 (1980). For a comprehensive review of the scientific literature on natural means of birth control, see Laurie Baillie, N.D., "Natural Birth Control," in Joseph E. Pizzorno and Michael T. Murray, *Textbook of Natural Medicine* (Seattle: Bastyr, John, College Publications, 1988).

31. P. Wharton et al., "Infertility in Male Pesticide Workers," *Lancet* (1977), pp. 1259–61; M. Donald Whorton et al., "Reproductive Hazards," chap. 20 in *Occupational Health: Recognizing and Preventing Work Related Disease*, ed. Barry S. Levy and David H. Wegman (Boston: Little Brown, 1983); R. E. Seegmiller et al., "Reporting of Congenital Malformations of Utah Birth Certificates," Utah Department of Health, April 1981; Colin Norman, "Vietnam's Herbicide Legacy," *Science* 219 (March 1, 1983); Council on Environmental Quality, *Chemical Hazards to Human Reproduction* (Washington D.C.: U.S. Government Printing Office, 1981); Christopher Norwood, "Terata," *Mother Jones* 10, no. 1 (January 1985), pp. 14–21.

32. Frances Moore Lappe and Joseph Collins, *World Hunger: Ten Myths*, 4th ed. (San Francisco: Institute for Food and Development, 1980). See also Chapter 4 for further discussion.

33. I am terming fertility problems as manmade epidemics when they are the result of toxic substances in the environment that are a consequence of thoughtless industrialization or the result of technologically advanced birth control devices such as the pill and IUD. Some female infertility problems today are the result of delayed childbearing, and I do not include such diversity-promoting life-cycle changes in the iatrogenic disease category.

Undoubtedly the degree of women centeredness and ecological consciousness fostered by practicing fertility awareness as a method of birth prevention will be shaped by a variety of factors—the values of the particular practitioner, her circle of friends and kin, her partners, where she lives, and the work she engages in on a daily basis. We know for example that in traditional societies or contemporary intentional communities where groups of women sleep together outdoors, undisturbed by any form of artificial light, the cycles of the entire group of women tend to converge with the twenty-eight day cycling of the moon. Contemporary practices of fertility awareness may be said to be an adaptation to cultural conditions where such group practices no longer obtain. The degree of ecological consciousness that fertility awareness fosters will also be influenced by a woman's involvement in some form of organic planting or other such seasonal activities. Working with the soil on a regular basis fosters awareness of the lunar cycles of plants. Of course in the contemporary industrialized world, women who self-consciously choose to become organic farmers will not need fertility awareness to make them ecologically conscious. At the same time, as a consequence of the ramifications of our modern language of control, women who already work with the soil may well need training in how to read their particular cycles. And among women whose bodies have been depleted because of inadequate nutrition (whether induced through man-made calamities or patriarchal women-hating practices), the "natural" reading of bodily signs may be neither simple or possible. Fertility awareness will not rectify the ravages of modern technical civilization through miracles. For a discussion of the lunar cycle and the menstrual cycles, see Shaffii and Shaffi, eds., *Biological Rhythms, Mood Disorders, Light Therapy, and the Pineal Gland* (Washington, D.C.: American Psychiatric Press: 1990), chap. 7. See also Janet Daling et al., "Primary Tubal Infertility in Relation to the Use of an Intrauterine Device," in *The New England Journal of Medicine*, no. 312 (April 11, 1985).

34. Angus MacLaren, *Reproductive Rituals* (London: Methuen, 1984). I should be clear here that I am not trying to create a new norm around fertility awareness as a method of birth prevention. My goal is simply to open up what we take into account when we think of matters of fertility and sensuality. I find Mira Sadgopal's concept of "fertility friendly" practices useful. Hormonal implants, pills, and pregnancy vaccines would be considered less

friendly than fertility awareness, diaphragms, and condoms. Decisions about what is most appropriate must of course be made by individual users.

35. Catharine MacKinnon, *Feminism Unmodified: Discourses on Life and Law* (Cambridge: Harvard University Press, 1987): "My stance is that the abortion choice must be legally available and must be *women's,* but not because the fetus is not a form of life. In the usual argument, the abortion decision is made contingent on whether the fetus is a form of life. I cannot follow that. Why should women not make life and death decisions?"

36. Ibid., p. 102.

37. Celia Wolfe-Devine, "Is Support for Abortion Essential to Feminism?" *New Oxford Review* (November 1990), p. 12.

38. While I am skeptical of the pro-choice view that better planning would eliminate the need for abortion I am equally skeptical of another variant of the pro-choice position which suggests an almost invariant need for abortion. In my view a culture that promotes social isolation and glorifies coercive sex will likely generate a higher demand for abortion than one in which women command respect and the multifold nature of pleasure and desire is acknowledged. A culture and mode of production that routinely generates environmental disasters and lock-step career patterns will also generate a higher demand for abortion. At the same time the use of contraceptive techniques that do not require the erasure of women's cycles and may be said to be fertility friendly, may sometimes increase the need for abortion.

CHAPTER 4
Children without Turmoil

1. Phillip Elmer-Dewitt, "Making Babies," *Time* (Sept. 30, 1991), p. 44.

2. Ibid., p. 45.

3. Michel Foucault, *History of Sexuality,* vol. 1 (New York: Pantheon, 1978), p. 143.

4. Ibid., pp. 146–47.

5. Jean Bethke Elshtain, "Technology as Destiny: The New Eugenics Challenges Feminism," *The Progressive* (June 1989), pp. 19–23.

6. Janice C. Raymond, "International Traffic in Reproduction," *Ms.* (May/June 1991), pp. 28–33.

7. Lori Andrews, *Between Strangers: Surrogate Mothers, Expectant Fathers, and Brave New Babies* (New York: Harper and Row, 1989), p. 159, as quoted in Dr. Jocelynne A. Scott, "Book Reviews," *Reproductive and Genetic Engineering: Journal of International Feminist Analysis* 3, no. 1 (1990), p. 74.

8. Ibid.

9. Raymond, "International Traffic in Reproduction," p. 32.

10. David Kaplan, "Equal Rights, Equal Risks: Women Are Now Free to Choose Dangerous Jobs," *Newsweek,* April 1, 1991.

11. Ruth Rosen, *New York Times,* April 1, 1991, p. A24.

12. Barbara Katz Rothman, *The Tentative Pregnancy* (New York: Viking, 1986).

13. See George J. Annas, "Is a Genetic Screening Test Ready When the Lawyers Say It Is?" *Hastings Center Report* (December 1985), pp. 16–18; and Robert Steinbrook, "In California, Voluntary Mass Prenatal Screening," *Hastings Center Report* (October 1986), pp. 4–7.

14. Steinbrook, "In California," p. 6.

15. Ruth Hubbard, "Personal Courage Is Not Enough," in *Test-Tube Women: What Future for Motherhood,* ed. Rita Arditti, Renata Duelli Klein, and Shelly Minden (London: Pandora Press, 1984), p. 350.

16. Anne Finger, "Claiming All of Our Bodies: Reproductive Rights and Disabilities," and Marsha Saxton, "Born and Unborn: The Implications of Reproductive Technologies for People with Disabilities," in *Test-Tube Women,* ed. Rita Arditti, Renata Duelli Klein, and Shelly Minden; and Adrienne Asch and Michelle Fined, "Shared Dreams: A Left Perspective on Disability Rights and Reproductive Rights," *Radical America* 18 (1984), pp. 51–58.

17. *Issues in Reproductive and Genetic Engineering: Journal of International Feminist Analysis* devotes itself to this sort of research.

18. Certainly what is commonly referred to as the "turkey baster method," in which male sperm is donated, does not rely on the medical or legal establishment. More commonly we find an increasing array of regulations to monitor access and protect donors and clients. As a consequence, when artificial insemination with frozen A.I.D.S.-free semen is successful it is rarely the result of a simple procedure. More often than not it will require several attempts and will have involved the use of fertility drugs whose full consequences we have yet to discern.

19. Note, "Reproductive Technology and the Procreative Rights of the Unmarried," *Harvard Law Review* 98 (January 1985), p. 685.

20. John Postage, "Bat's Chance in Hell," *New Scientist* 58 (April 5, 1973), p. 16, as cited by Christine Overall, *Ethics and Human Reproduction* (Boston: Allen and Unwin, 1987), p. 29.

21. Carl J. Bajema, "The Genetic Implications of American Lifestyles in Reproduction and Population Control," in *Population, Environment, and People,* ed. Noel Hinrichs (New York: McGraw-Hill, 1971), p. 70.

22. Bentley Glass, "Science: Endless Horizons or Golden Age?" *Science* 171 (1971), pp. 21–29, as cited in Hubbard, "Personal Courage."

23. John A. Robertson, "Procreative Liberty and the Control of Conception, Pregnancy, and Childbirth," *Virginia Law Review* 69 (1983), p. 450.

24. Aubrey Milunsky, *Genetic Disorders and the Fetus* (New York: Plenum Press, 1986), p. 11.

25. Cynthia R. Daniels, *At Women's Expense: State Power and the Politics of Fetal Rights* (Cambridge: Harvard University Press, 1993).

26. Cynthia R. Daniels, "Pregnancy and Self-Sovereignty: State Power and Fetal Animation," paper presented at the Annual Meeting of the Western Political Science Association, Pasadena, California, March 1993.

27. Ibid.

28. Darlene Johnson appealed the judge's condition of probation and, as of May 15, 1992, was not forced to use Norplant. See also, for example, Marlene Gerber Fried and Loretta Ross, "'Our Bodies, Our Lives: Our Right to Decide': The Struggle for Abortion Rights and Reproductive Freedom," *Radical America* 24, no. 2 (1992), pp. 31–37; Janet Gallagher, "What is Wrong With Fetal Rights," *Harvard Women's Law Journal* (1987).

29. Marlene Gerber Fried and Loretta Ross, "Reproductive Rights Under Siege," *Radical America* 24, no. 2, n.d., p. 32.

30. John Horgan, "Eugenics Revisited," *Scientific American* (June 1993), p. 123. This is an invaluable article which reviews the dubious links between genes and behavior.

31. Irwin Chargaff, "Engineering a Molecular Nightmare," *Nature* 329 (May 1987), p. 199.

32. See Rosalie Bertell, *No Immediate Danger: Prognosis for a Radioactive Earth* (London: The Women's Press, 1987), for a discussion of the health effects of radiation exposure.

33. Tom Muir and Anne Sudar, "Toxic Chemicals in the Great Lakes Basin Ecosystem—Some Observations" (Burlington, Ontario:

Water Planning and Management Branch, Inland Waters/Land Directorate, Ontario Region, November 1987), provides a valuable overview of ecosystem contamination as it affects human and nonhuman reproduction. See also Colborn and Clement, eds., *Chemically-Induced Alterations in Sexual and Functional Development: The Wildlife/Human Connection* (Princeton: Princeton Scientific Publishing, 1992).

CHAPTER 5

Food without Sweat

1. Aldous Huxley, *Brave New World Revisited* (New York: Bantam, 1958).
2. Wendell Berry, *The Unsettling of America: Culture and Agriculture* (New York: Avon, 1977), p. 58.
3. See, for example, Marshall Sahlins, *Stone Age Economics* (Chicago: Aldine, 1972).
4. Nicholas Xenos, *Scarcity and Modernity* (New York: Routledge, 1989), p. 35.
5. And it has been the principle means by which the bones of "primitive" and "exotic" peoples have been stolen from sacred burial sites and placed in the sealed halls of Western museums and archaeological institutions. See, for example, "Native Americans versus Archaeologists: The Legal Issues," *American Indian Law Review* 10 (1982), pp. 91–93.
6. Gustavo Estera, "The Modernization of Poverty," *The Indian Express* (January 4, 1992), p. 5. The quote from Truman is taken from this article.
7. Berry, *Unsettling of America,* p. 136.
8. Alan B. Durning and Holly B. Brough, *Taking Stock: Animal Farming and the Environment,* World Watch Paper 103 (July 1991). See especially pp. 19–20.
9. Ruth Schwartz Cowan, *More Work for Mother: The Ironies of Household Technology from the Open Hearth to the Microwave* (New York: Basic Books, 1983), p. 53.
10. Ibid., p. 66.
11. Berry, *Unsettling of America,* p. 33.
12. Cary Fowler and Pat Mooney, *Shattering: Food Politics and the Loss of Genetic Diversity* (Tucson: University of Arizona Press, 1990), p. 47.
13. For a discussion, see, for example, A. Westling, ed., *Envi-*

ronmental Warfare: A Technical, Legal and Policy Appraisal (London: Taylor and Francis, 1984).

14. Fowler and Mooney, *Shattering,* p. 177. See also Alfred Crosby, *Ecological Imperialism: The Biological Expansion of Europe 900–1900* (Cambridge: Cambridge University Press, 1986).

15. As quoted in Susan George, *Ill Fares the Land: Essays on Food, Hunger, and Power* (Washington D.C.: Institute for Policy Studies, 1984), p. 22.

16. See, for example, Gita Sen and Caren Grown, *Development, Crises, and Alternative Visions: Third World Women's Perspectives* (New York: Monthly Review Press, 1987).

17. Vandana Shiva, *Staying Alive: Women, Ecology, and Development* (London: Zed Press, 1988), p. 61.

18. Ibid., p. 219.

19. Carolyn Merchant, in *Ecological Revolutions: Nature, Gender, and Science in New England* (Chapel Hill: University of North Carolina Press, 1989), p. 63, observes, "In the struggle to set humans apart from nature, Puritans, like Europeans, soon outlawed human sex with animals, making "bestiality" (or buggery) a capital crime for males."

20. John S. Aird, *Slaughter of the Innocents* (Washington, D.C.: The AEI Press, 1990), p. 20.

21. Michel Foucault, *The History of Sexuality,* vol. 1 (New York: Pantheon, 1978), p. 25.

22. Barbara Duden, "Population," in Wolfgang Sachs, *The Development Dictionary: A Guide to Knowledge and Power* (London: Zed Press, 1991), p. 148.

23. Wangari Maathai, *The Green Belt Movement* (Nairobi: Environmental Liaison Centre International, 1988), pp. 1–31.

24. Fowler and Mooney, *Shattering,* p. 77.

25. Usha Menon, "Intellectual Property Rights and Agricultural Development," *Economic and Political Weekly* 26, nos. 27 and 28 (July 6–13 1991), pp. 1660–67; and Henk Hobbelink, *Biotechnology and the Future of World Agriculture: The Fourth Resource* (London: Zed, 1991).

26. Anvil Agarwal and Sunita Narain, *Global Warming in an Unequal World: A Case of Environmental Colonization* (New Delhi: Centre for Science and Environment, 1991).

27. Maria Mies, assisted by Lalita K. and Krishna Kumari, *Indian Women in Subsistence and Agricultural Labour,* Women Work and Development Monograph #12 (Geneva: International Labour Organisation, 1986), p. 114.

28. Pam Simmons, "Women in Development a Threat to Liberation," *The Ecologist* 22, no. 1 (January/February 1992), p. 19.
29. See Betsy Hartmann, *Reproductive Rights and Wrongs* (New York: Harper and Row, 1987), pp. 126–43, for a discussion of what she terms "the 'new look.'"
30. "New Draft Plan for Family Planning," *Indian Express,* January 4, 1992, p. A1.
31. Bina Agarwal, "Neither Sustenance nor Sustainability," in *Structures of Patriarchy: The State, the Community, and the Household in Modernising Asia* (London: Zed, 1988), p. 110.
32. It is important to note here the rapid shift of discourse within the development community in the post-Brundtland era where development has been linked to concern for the environment. As the poor are identified as the agents of destruction and as women are identified as victims of environmental degradation, development objectives now increasingly focus on helping women to improve their skills as "resource managers." For an insightful critique of the new consensus of women, population, and environment, see Betsy Hartmann, "Old Maps and New Terrains: The Politics of Women, Population, and the Environment," paper presented at The Fifth International Interdisciplinary Congress on Women, San Jose, Costa Rica, February 23, 1993.
33. Shive, *Staying Alive,* p. 113.
34. Forum Against Sex Determination and Sex Pre-selection, "Campaign Against Sex Determination and Sex Pre-Selection in India: Our Experience" (Bombay: Women's Centre, n.d.).

CHAPTER 6

Our Bodies, Our Earth

1. "Global Management," *The Ecologist* 22, no. 3 (July/August), p. 180.
2. For a critique of the whole Earth image, see Yaakov Jerome Garb, "Perspective or Escape? Ecofeminist Musings on Contemporary Earth Imagery," in *Reweaving the World" The Emergence of Ecofeminism,* ed. Irene Diamond and Gloria Feman Orenstein (San Francisco: Sierra Club, 1990), pp. 264–78.
3. Gopal Guru, "Laxmi Mukti," *Economic and Political Weekly* (July 1992); Gail Omvedt, "Laxmi Mukti," *Hitavada* (December 27, 1992).
4. See Ilina Sen, ed., *A Space Within the Struggle: Women's Par-*

ticipation in People's Movements (New Delhi: Kali for Women, 1990); Gail Omvedt, "The Awakening of Women's Power: The Rural Women's Movement in India," unpublished manuscript, 1992.

5. For a critique of the Brundtland Report and sustainable development, see Shiv Visvanathan, "Mrs. Brundtland's Disenchanted Cosmos," *Alternatives* "Social Transformation and Humane Governance 16, no. 3 (Summer 1991), pp. 377–84.

6. My discussion of global managers and their effort to further enclose the commons throughout this chapter draws heavily on the special issue of *The Ecologist,* vol. 22, no. 4 (July/August 1992), entitled "Whose Common Future?"

7. Lois Gibbs, as told to Murray Levine, *Love Canal: My Story* (Albany: State University Press of New York, 1982); Rachel Bagby, "Daughters of Growing Things," in Diamond and Orenstein, eds., *Reweaving the World;* Wangari Maathai, *The Greenbelt Movement* (Nairobi, Environmental Liaison Centre International, 1988); interview with Medha Patkar, *India International Center Quarterly 1990* 19, nos. 1–2 (Spring/Summer 1992), pp. 273–99.

8. Teresa Santa Clara Gomes, "A Feminine Utopia," in *Terra Femina,* p. 89.

9. See Starhawk, "Power, Authority, and Mystery: Ecofeminism and Earth-based Spirituality," in Diamond and Orenstein, eds., *Reweaving the World,* p. 79, for a discussion of Greenham Common.

10. For a discussion of this march, see "Break-through despite Break-up: Protect Waters! Protect Life!," Kanya Humari March, National Fisherman's Forum, Cochin, October 10, 1989.

11. For a critique of the canonical view of evolution that reinforces human superiority, see Stephen Jay Gould, *Wonderful Life: The Burgess Shale and the Nature of History* (New York: Norton, 1989).

12. Jane Bennett, *Unthinking Faith and Enlightenment* (New York: New York University Press, 1989), p. 158.

13. Excellent sources for reports on such community efforts are *The Utne Reader, Catalyst, The New Catalyst,* and *Rain* magazine; see especially the *Rain* issue on "Working Communities," vol. 14, no. 2 (Winter/Spring 1992); on the possibilities of barter exchange, see Michell Silver, "The Ultimate Barter," *Mother Earth News* (August/September 1993); on bioregional approaches to economics see Susan Meeker Lowry, *Economics as if the Earth Really Mattered* (Philadelphia: New Society Publishers, 1988).

14. Thomas Kuehl, "The Nature of the State: An Ecological Rereading of Sovereignty and Territory," in *Reimagining the Nation* (London: Open University Press, forthcoming).

15. Madhu Kishwar, *Gandhi and Women* (New Delhi: Manushi Prakashan, 1986), p. 2.

AFTERWORD
Coming to Rest

1. Garret Hardin, *Living Within Limits* (New York: Oxford University Press, 1993).

2. Abraham Joshua Heschel, *The Sabbath* (New York: Farrar, Straus and Giroux, 1951), p. 28.

3. Henry Abramovitch, "Death," in Arthur A. Cohen and Paul Mendes-Flohr, eds., *Contemporary Jewish Religious Thought* (New York: Charles Scribners, 1987), p. 132.

4. "Tumah and taharah-mikveh," in Richard Siegal, Michael Strassfeld, and Sharon Strassfeld, eds., *The First Jewish Catalogue* (Philadelphia: Jewish Publication Society of America, 1973), pp. 167–71.

5. Arthur Waskow, "Rest," in Cohen and Mendes-Flohr, eds., *Contemporary Jewish Religious Thought*, p. 805.

SELECT
BIBLIOGRAPHY

ADAMS, CAROL J., ed. *Ecofeminism and the Sacred*. New York: Continuum Publishing Co., 1993.

AGARWAL, ANIL and SUNITA NARAIN. *Global Warming in an Unequal World: A Case of Environmental Colonization*. New Delhi: Centre for Science and Environment, 1991.

AGARWAL, ANIL, et al. *The Fight for Survival: People's Action for Environment*. New Delhi: Centre for Science and Development, 1987.

AGARWAL, BINA. "Neither Sustenance nor Sustainability." In *Structures of Patriarchy: The State, the Community, and the Household in Modernising Asia*, edited by Bina Agarwal. London: Zed Books, 1988.

AKHTER, FARIDA. *Depopulating Bangladesh*. Dhaka, Bangladesh: Ubinig, 1986.

ALLEN, PAULA GUNN. *The Sacred Hoop: Recovering the Feminine in American Indian Traditions*. Boston: Beacon Press, 1986.

ANNAS, GEORGE J. "Is a Genetic Screening Test Ready When the Lawyers Say It Is?" *Hastings Center Report* (December 1985), pp. 16–18.

APFEL, R.J., and S. M. FISCHER. *DES and the Dilemmas of Modern Medicine*. New Haven: Yale University Press, 1984.

ARDITTI, RITA, RENATA DUELLI KLEIN, and SHELLY MINDEN, eds. *Test-Tube Women: What Future for Motherhood?* London: Pandora Press, 1984.

ARENDT, HANNAH. *The Human Condition*. Chicago: University of Chicago Press, 1958.

ASCH, ADRIENNE, and MICHELLE FIND. "Shared Dreams: A Left

Perspective on Disability Rights and Reproductive Rights." *Radical America* 18 (1984): 51–58.

BAJEMA, CARL J. "The Genetic Implications of American Lifestyles in Reproduction and Population Control." In *Population, Environment, and People,* edited by Noel Hinrichs. New York: Ballantine Books, 1991.

BEINFIELD, HARRIET, AND EFREM KORNGOLD. *Between Heaven and Earth: A Guide to Chinese Medicine.* New York: Ballantine Books, 1991.

BENNETT, JANE. *Unthinking Faith and Enlightenment: Nature and the State in a Post-Hegelian Era.* New York: New York University Press, 1987.

BERRY, WENDELL. *The Gift of Good Land: Further Essays, Cultural and Agricultural.* San Francisco: North Point Press, 1981.

———. *The Unsettling of American: Culture and Agriculture.* New York: Avon, 1977.

———. *Home Economics.* San Francisco: North Point Press, 1987.

BIEHL, JANET. *Rethinking Ecofeminist Politics.* Boston: South End Press, 1991.

BIGWOOD, CAROL. *Earth Muse: Feminism, Nature, and Art.* Philadelphia: Temple University Press, 1993.

BOTKIN, DANIEL B. *Discordant Harmonies: A New Ecology for the Twenty-First Century.* New York: Oxford University Press, 1990.

BUVINIC, MAYRA, MARGARET A. LYCETTE, AND WILLIAM PAUL McGREEVEY, EDS. *Women and Poverty in the Third World.* Baltimore: Johns Hopkins University Press, 1982.

CALDECOTT, LEONIE, AND STEPHANIE LELAND, EDS. *Reclaim the Earth: Women Speak Out for Life on Earth.* London: The Women's Press, 1983

"Campaign Against Sex Determination and Sex Pre-Selection in India: Our Experience." Bombay: Women's Centre, undated.

CHARA, R. ALTA. "Medicine and the Law: Mandatory Contraception," *The Lancét* 339 (May 1992), pp. 1104–5.

CHARGAFF, IRWIN. "Engineering a Molecular Nightmare." *Nature* 329 (May 1987), p. 199.

CHAYANIKA, SWATIJI, AND KAMAXI. *We and Our Fertility.* Bombay: Research Centre for Women's Studies, 1990.

CHRIST, CAROL P. *The Laughter of Aphrodite: Reflections on a Journey to the Goddess.* San Francisco: Harper and Row, 1987.

CODE, LORRAINE. *What Can She Know? Feminist Theory and the Construction of Knowledge.* Ithaca: Cornell University Press, 1991.

COLBURN, THEO, FREDERICK S. VOM SAAL, AND ANA M. SOTO. "Developmental Effects of Endocrine-Disrupting Chemicals in Wildlife and Humans," *Environmental Health Perspectives* 101, no. 5 (October 1993), pp. 378–84.

COLLARD, ANDREE, WITH JOYCE CONTRUCCI. *The Rape of the Wild: Man's Violence Against Animals and the Earth.* Bloomington: Indiana University Press, 1989.

COOK, ALICE, AND GWYN KIRK. *Greenham Common Women Everywhere.* London: South End, 1983.

COREA, GENA, ET AL. *Man-Made Women: How New Reproductive Technologies Affect Women.* Bloomington: Indiana University Press, 1987.

COREA, GENA. *The Mother Machine: Reproductive Technologies from Artificial Insemination to Artificial Wombs.* New York: Harper and Row, Perennial Library, 1985.

CORNELL, DRUCILLA. *Beyond Accommodation.* New York: Routledge, 1991.

Council on Environmental Quality. *Chemical Hazards to Human Reproduction.* Washington D.C.: U.S. Government Printing Office, 1981.

COWAN, RUTH SCHWARTZ. *More Work for Mother: The Ironies of Household Technology from the Open Hearth to the Microwave.* New York: Basic Books, 1983.

D'EAUBONNE, FRANCOISE. "Feminism or Death." In *New French Feminisms,* edited by Elaine Marks and Isabelle de Courtivron. New York: Schocken, 1981.

DALY, MARY. *Gyn/Ecology, the Metaethics of Radical Feminism.* Boston: Beacon Press, 1978.

DE BEAUVOIR, SIMONE. *The Second Sex.* Translated and edited by H. M. Parshley. New York: Alfred A. Knopf, 1952.

DE OLIVEIRA, ROSISKA DARCY. "Women and Nature: An Ancestral Bond, a New Alliance." In *Terra Femina,* edited by Rosiska Darcy de Oliveira and Thais Corral. Rio de Janeiro: REDEH, 1992.

DE OLIVEIRA, ROSISKA DARCY, THAIS CORRAL, AND FATIMA VIANNA MELLO. *Population Danger: Sex, Lies, and Misconceptions.* Rio de Janeiro: IDAC/REDEH/IBASE, 1993.

Development for Whom? A Critique of Women's Development Programmes. New Delhi: Saheli, 1991.

Development Where Nature, Women and Men Matter: Tenth Year Review. Trivandarum: Community Development Corporation, n.d.

DIAMOND, IRENE, AND GLORIA FEMAN ORENSTEIN, EDS. *Reweaving the World: The Emergence of Ecofeminism.* San Francisco: Sierra Club, 1990.

DIETRICH, GABRIELE. *Women's Movement in India.* Bangalore, India: Breakthrough Publications, 1988.

DOUGHERTY, JAMES. "Jane Addams: Culture and Imagination." *Yale Review* (April 1982), pp. 367–68.

DURNING, ALAN B., AND HOLLY B. BROUGH. "Taking Stock: Animal Farming and the Environment." *World Watch Paper* 103 (July 1991), pp. 19–20.

ELMER-DEWITT, PHILLIP. "Making Babies." *Time* (Sept. 30, 1991), p. 44.

ELSHTAIN, JEAN BETHKE. "Technology as Destiny: The New Eugenics Challenges Feminism." *The Progressive* (June 1989), pp. 19–23.

ESTEVA, GUSTAVO. "The Modernisation of Poverty." *The Indian Express* (January 4, 1992), p. 5.

EURIPIDES. *The Bacchae.* Translated by Michael Cacoyannis. New York: New American Library, 1982.

FALK, MARCIA. *Love Lyrics From the Bible: A Translation and Literary Study of the Song of Songs.* Sheffield, England: The Almond Press, 1982.

———. "Notes on Composing New Blessings."

FERGUSON, KATHY. *The Man Question: Visions of Subjectivity in Feminist Theory.* Berkeley: University of California Press, 1993.

FINGER, ANNE. "Claiming All of Our Bodies: Reproductive Rights and Disabilities." In *Test-Tube Women,* edited by Rita Arditti, Renata Duelli Klein, and Shelly Minden. London: Pandora Press, 1984.

FIRESTONE, SHULAMITH. *Dialectic of Sex: The Case for Feminist Revolution.* New York: Bantam Books, 1971.

FLAX, JANE. *Thinking Fragments: Psychoanalysis, Feminism, and Postmodernism in the Contemporary West.* Berkeley: University of California Press, 1990.

FOUCAULT, MICHEL. *The History of Sexuality,* vol. 1. Translated by Robert Hurley. New York: Pantheon Books, 1978.

———. *Foucault Live (Interviews, 1966–84).* New York: Semiotext(e), 1989.

———. *Power/Knowledge: Selected Interviews and Other Writ-*

ings, 1972–1977. Edited by Colin Gordon. New York: Pantheon Books, 1980.

———. "The Subject and Power." In *Michel Foucault: Beyond Structuralism and Hermeneutics,* edited by Hubert L. Dreyfus and Paul Rabinow. Chicago: University of Chicago Press, 1982.

FOWLER, CARY, AND PAT MOONEY. *Shattering: Food, Politics and the Loss of Genetic Diversity.* Tucson: University of Arizona Press, 1990.

FOX, MICHAEL W. *Agricide: The Hidden Crisis that Affects Us All.* New York: Schocken, 1986.

FRENCH, HILARY F. *Costly Tradeoffs: Reconciling Trade and the Environment.* Washington D.C.: Worldwatch Paper 113, March 1993.

FRIED, MARLENE GERBER, AND LORETTA ROSS. "'Our Bodies, Our Lives: Our Right to Decide': The Struggle for Abortion Rights and Reproductive Freedom." *Radical America* 24, no. 2 (1992), pp. 31–37.

GAARD, GRETA, ED. *Ecofeminism: Women, Animals, Nature.* Philadelphia: Temple University Press, 1993.

GARB, YAAKOV JEROME. "Perspective or Escape? Ecofeminist Musings on Contemporary Earth Imagery." In *Reweaving the World: The Emergence of Ecofeminism,* edited by Irene Diamond and Gloria Feman Orenstein. San Francisco: Sierra Club, 1990.

GELPI, BARBARA C., ED. *Women and Poverty.* Chicago: University of Chicago Press, 1986.

GEORGE, SUSAN. *Ill Fares the Land: Essays on Food, Hunger, and Power.* Washington D.C.: Institute for Policy Studies, 1984.

———. *A Fate Worse than Debt.* London: Penguin, 1988.

GILLIGAN, CAROL. *In a Different Voice: Psychological Theory and Women's Development.* Cambridge: Harvard University Press, 1982.

GIMBUTAS, MARIJA. *The Goddesses and Gods of Old Europe, 6500–3500 B.C.: Myths, Legends, and Cult Images.* Berkeley: University of California Press, 1982.

GLASS, BENTLEY. "Science: Endless Horizons or Golden Age?" *Science* 171 (1971), pp. 21–29.

GOLDENBERG, NAOMI R. *Returning Words to Flesh: Feminism, Psychoanalysis, and the Resurrection of the Body.* Boston: Beacon Press, 1990.

GOLDSMITH, EDWARD. *The Way: An Ecological World-View.* Boston: Shambhala, 1993.

GOMEZ, TERESA SANTA CLARA. "A Feminine Utopia." In *Terra Femina,* p. 89.

GORDON, LINDA. *Woman's Body, Woman's Right,* 2d ed. New York: Penguin, 1990.

GOULD, STEPHEN J. *This Wonderful Life.* New York: Norton, 1989.

GRAY, ELIZABETH DODSON. *Green Paradise Lost.* Wellesley, Mass.: Roundtable Press, 1981.

GREER, GERMAINE. *Sex and Destiny: The Politics of Human Fertility.* New York: Harper and Row, 1984.

GRIFFIN, SUSAN. *Made From This Earth.* London: Women's Press, 1982.

———. *Woman and Nature: The Roaring Inside Her.* San Francisco: Harper and Row, 1978.

———. *Pornography and Silence: Culture's Revenge Against Nature.* New York: Harper and Row, 1981.

GUHA, RAMACHANDRA. *The Unquiet Woods: Ecological Change and Peasant Resistance in the Himalaya.* Delhi: Oxford University Press, 1989.

GURU, GOPAL. "Shetkari Sanghtana and the Pursuit of 'Laxmi Mukti'." *Economic and Political Weekly* (July 1992), pp. 1463–1465.

HAMILTON, CYNTHIA. "Women, Home, and Community: The Struggle in an Urban Environment." In *Reweaving the World: the Emergence of Ecofeminism,* edited by Irene Diamond and Gloria Feman Orenstein. San Francisco: Sierra Club, 1990.

HANCOCK, GRAHAM. *Lords of Poverty: The Power, Prestige, and Corruption of the International Aid Business.* New York: Atlantic Monthly Press, 1989.

HARAWAY, DONNA. "A Manifesto for Cyborgs: Science, Technology, and Socialist Feminism in the 1980s." *Socialist Review* 80 (1985), pp. 65–107.

———. "Situated Knowledges: The Science Question in Feminism and the Privilege of Partial Perspective." *Feminist Studies* 14, no. 3 (Fall 1988).

HARDING, SANDRA, AND MERRILL B. HINTIKKA, EDS. *Discovering Reality: Feminist Perspectives on Epistemology, Metaphysics, Methodology, and Philosophy of Science.* Dordrecht, Holland: D. Reidel, 1983.

HARRIS, ADRIENNE, AND YNESTRA KING, EDS. *Rocking the Ship of State: Toward a Feminist Peace Politics.* Boulder: Westview Press, 1989.

HARTMANN, BETSY. *Reproductive Rights and Wrongs: The Global Politics of Population Control and Contraceptive Choice.* New York: Harper and Row, 1987.

———. "Old Maps and New Terrain: The Politics of Women, Population, and the Environment in the 1990s," paper presented at the fifth International Interdisciplinary Congress of Women, San Jose, Costa Rica, February 1993.

HARTSOCK, NANCY C. M. *Money, Sex and Power: Toward a Feminist Historical Materialism.* New York: Longman, 1983.

HEINSOHN, GUNNAR, AND OTTO STEIGER. "The Elimination of Modern Birth Control and the Witch Trials of Modern Times." *International Journal of Women's Studies* 5, no. 3, n.d., pp. 193–214.

HERBST, A. L., AND H. A. BERNE. *Developmental Effects of Diethylstilbestrol (DES) in Pregnancy.* New York: Thieme Stratton, 1981.

HESCHEL, ABRAHAM. *The Sabbath: Its Meaning for Modern Man.* New York: Farrar, Straus, and Giroux, 1951.

HINRICHS, NOEL, ED. *Population, Environment, and People.* New York: McGraw-Hill, 1971.

HOBBELINK, HENK. *Biotechnology and the Future of World Agriculture: The Fourth Resource.* London: Zed, 1991.

HODGSON, DENNIS. "The Ideological Origins of the Populations Association of America." *Population and Development Review,* no. 17 (March 1991), pp. 1–34.

HONIG, BONNIE. *Political Theory and the Displacement of Politics.* Ithaca: Cornell University Press, 1993.

HUBBARD, RUTH AND WALD, ELIJAH. *Exploding the Gene Myth: How Genetic Information Is Produced and Manipulated by Scientists, Physicians, Employers, Insurance Companies, Educators, and Law Enforcers.* Boston: Beacon Press, 1993.

HUBBARD, RUTH. "Personal Courage Is Not Enough." In *Test-Tube Women: What Future for Motherhood,* edited by Rita Arditti, Renata Duelli Klein, and Shelly Minden. London: Pandora Press, 1984.

———. "Eugenics and Prenatal Testing." *International Journal of Health Services* 16, no. 2 (1986).

———. "Prenatal Diagnosis and Eugenic Ideology." *Women's Studies International Forum* 8 (1985).

HULSBERG, WERNER. *The German Greens: A Social and Political Profile.* Translated by Gus Fagan. London: Verso, 1988.

HUXLEY, ALDOUS. *Brave New World Revisited.* New York: Bantam, 1958.

HYDE, LEWIS. *The Gift: Imagination and the Erotic Life of Property.* New York: Random House, 1983.

Issues in Reproductive and Genetic Engineering: Journal of International Feminist Analysis.

JAIN, SHOBHITA. "Women and People's Ecological Movement: A Case Study of Women's Role in the Chipko Movement in Uttar Pradesh." *Economic and Political Weekly* 19, no. 41 (October 1984), pp. 1788–1794.

JANSSON, ERIK. "The Causes of Birth Defects, Learning Disabilities, and Mental Retardation in Relation to Laboratory Animal Testing Requirements and Needs." *National Network to Prevent Birth Defects News* (June 14, 1988).

JONAS, ROBERT A. "Birth Control in a Culture of Changing Sex Roles: The NFP Experience." Unpublished dissertation, Harvard Graduate School of Education, 1983.

JONES, LYNNE, ED. *Keeping the Peace.* London: Women's Press, 1983.

KELLER, CATHERINE. *From a Broken Web: Separation, Sexism and Self.* Boston: Beacon Press, 1986.

KELLER, EVELYN FOX, AND CHRISTINE R. GRONTKOWSKI. "The Mind's Eye." In *Discovering Reality: Feminist Perspectives on Epistemology, Metaphysics, Methodology, and Philosophy of Science,* edited by Sandra Harding and Merrill B. Hintikka. Dordrecht, Holland: D. Reidel, 1983.

KELLER, EVELYN FOX. *Reflections on Gender and Science.* New Haven, Conn.: Yale University Press, 1985.

KELLY, PETRA. *Fighting for Hope.* Translated by Marianne Howarth. Boston: South End Press, 1984.

———. *Nonviolence Speaks to Power.* Honolulu: Center for Global Nonviolence Planning Project, 1992.

KISHWAR, MADHU. *Gandhi and Women.* New Delhi: Manushi Prakashan, 1986.

KLEIN, RENATA DUELLI. "What's 'New' about the 'New' Reproductive Technologies?" In *Man-Made Women,* edited by Gena Corea et al. Bloomington: Indiana University Press, 1987.

KLOPPENBURG, JACK RALPH, JR. *First the Seed: The Political Economy of Plant Biotechnology, 1492–2000.* Cambridge: Cambridge University Press, 1988.

KRAEMER, ROSS SHEPARD. *Her Share of the Blessings.* Oxford: Oxford University Press, 1992.

LAPPE, FRANCES MOORE, AND JOSEPH COLLINS. *World Hunger: Ten Myths.* 4th ed. San Francisco: Institute for Food and Development, 1980.

LE GUIN, URSULA. *Always Coming Home.* New York: Harper, 1985.

LEACH, WILLIAM. *True Love and Perfect Union.* New York: Basic Books, 1980.

LEDERER, LAURA, ED. *Take Back the Night: Women and Pornography.* New York: William Morrow, 1980.

LEIDHOLDT, DORCHEN, AND JANICE G. RAYMOND, EDS. *The Sexual Liberals and the Attack on Feminism.* New York: Pergamon Press, The Athene Series, 1990.

LEMONS, J. STANLEY. *The Woman Citizen: Social Feminism in the 1920s.* Urbana: University of Illinois Press, 1973.

LORDE, AUDRE. *Sister Outsider: Essays and Speeches.* Trumansburg, N.Y.: Crossing Press, 1984.

LUKER, KIRSTEN. *Abortion and the Politics of Motherhood.* Berkeley: University of California Press, 1984.

MAATHAI, WANGARI. *The Green Belt Movement.* Nairobi: Environmental Liaison Centre International, 1988.

MACKINNON, CATHARINE A. *Feminism Unmodified: Discourses on Life and Law.* Cambridge, Mass.: Harvard University Press, 1987.

———. "Sexual Pornography and Method: Pleasure Under Patriarchy,," *Ethics* 99 (January 1989).

MACNEILL, JIM, PETER WINSEMIUS, AND TAIZO YAKUSHIJI, EDS. *Beyond Interdependence: The Meshing of the World's Economy and the Earth's Ecology.* New York: Oxford University Press, 1991.

MALTHUS, THOMAS ROBERT. *An Essay on the Principle of Population.* New York: Norton, 1976.

MAMDANI, MAHMOOD. *The Myth of Population Control: Family, Caste & Class in an Indian Village.* New York: Monthly Review Press, 1972.

MARTIN, EMILY. *The Woman in the Body: A Cultural Analysis of Reproduction.* Boston: Beacon Press, 1987.

MASS, BONNIE. *Population Target: The Political Economy of Population Control in Latin America.* Toronto: Women's Press, 1976.

MCALLISTER, PAM. *Reweaving the Web of Life: Feminism and Nonviolence.* Philadelphia: New Society, 1982.

McMILLAN, CAROL. *Women, Reason and Nature.* Princeton: Princeton University Press, 1982.

MENON, USHA. "Intellectual Property Rights and Agricultural Development." *Economic and Political Weekly* 26, nos. 27 and 28 (July 6–13, 1991), pp. 1660–1667.

MERCHANT, CAROLYN. *The Death of Nature; Women, Ecology and the Scientific Revolution.* New York: Harper and Row, 1980.

———. *Ecological Revolutions: Nature, Gender, and Science in New England.* Chapel Hill: University of North Carolina Press, 1989.

MIES, MARIA, ASSISTED BY LALITA K. AND KRISHNA KUMARI. "Indian Women in Subsistence and Agricultural Labour." *Women, Work and Development* 12. Geneva: International Labour Organisation, 1986.

MIES, MARIA. *Patriarchy and Accumulation on a World Scale: Women in the International Division of Labor.* London: Atlantic Highlands, 1986.

MILUNSKY, AUBREY. *Genetic Disorders and the Fetus.* New York: Plenum Press, 1986.

MITCHELL, JULIET. *Woman's Estate.* New York: Pantheon Books, 1971.

MOHR, JAMES C. *Abortion in America: the Origins and Evolutions of National Policy.* New York: Oxford University Press, 1978.

MUIR, TOM, AND ANNE SUDAR. "Toxic Chemicals in the Great Lakes Basin Ecosystem—Some Observations." Burlington, Ontario: Water Planning and Management Branch, Inland Waters/Land Directorate, Ontario Region, Canada, November 1987.

MUMFORD, LEWIS. *Technics and Civilization.* New York: Harcourt, Brace & Co., 1934.

NABHAN, GARY PAUL. *Enduring Seeds: Native American Agriculture and Wild Plant Conservation.* San Francisco: North Point Press, 1989.

"Native American versus Archaeologists: The Legal Issues." *American Indian Law Review* 10 (1982), pp. 91–93.

NORBERG-HODGE, HELENA. *Ancient Futures: Learning from Ladakh.* San Francisco: Sierra Club, 1991.

NORMAN, COLIN. "Vietnam's Herbicide Legacy." *Science* 219 (March 1, 1983).

NORWOOD, CHRISTOPHER. "Terata." *Mother Jones* 10, no. 1 (January 1985), pp. 14–21.

NORWOOD, VERA. *Made from this Earth*. Chapel Hill: University of North Carolina Press, 1993.

O'BRIEN, MARY. *The Politics of Reproduction*. Boston: Routledge and Kegan Paul, 1981.

OMVEDT, GAIL. "The Awakening of Women's Power: The Rural Women's Movement in India." Unpublished manuscript, 1992.

OVERALL, CHRISTINE. *Ethics and Human Reproduction*. Boston: Allen and Unwin, 1987.

PETCHESKY, ROSALIND P. *Abortion and Women's Choice: The State, Sexuality, and Reproductive Freedom*. New York: Longman, 1984.

————. "Reproduction, Ethics and Public Policy: The Federal Sterilization Regulations." *Hastings Center Report* 9, no. 5 (October 1979).

PLANT, JUDITH. "Searching for Common Ground: Ecofeminism and Bioregionalism." In *Reweaving the World: the Emergence of Ecofeminism*, edited by Irene Diamond and Gloria Feman Orenstein. San Francisco: Sierra Club, 1990.

PLASKOW, JUDITH, AND CAROL P. CHRIST, EDS. *Weaving the Visions: New Patterns in Feminist Spirituality*. San Francisco: Harper and Row, 1989.

PRENTICE, SUSAN. "Taking Sides: What's Wrong with Eco-Feminism?" *Women and Environments* 10, no. 3 (1988), pp. 9–10.

QUINBY, LEE. "Ecofeminism and the Politics of Resistance." In *Reweaving the World: the Emergence of Ecofeminism*, edited by Irene Diamond and Gloria Feman Orenstein.

RABINOW, PAUL, ED. *The Foucault Reader*. New York: Pantheon Books, 1984.

RAYMOND, JANICE C. "International Traffic in Reproduction." *Ms.* (May/June 1991), pp. 28–33.

REILLY, PHILIP P. *The Surgical Solution: A History of Involuntary Sterilization in the U.S.* Baltimore: Johns Hopkins, 1991.

"Reproductive Rights Under Siege." *Radical America* 24, no. 2, n.d., pp. 32–33.

"Reproductive Technology and the Procreative Rights of the Unmarried." *Harvard Law Review* 98 (January 1985), p. 685.

RICH, ADRIENNE. *Blood, Bread, and Poetry: Selected Prose 1979–1985*. New York: Norton, 1986.

————. *Of Woman Born*. New York: Bantam Books, 1976.

RIDDLE, JOHN M. *Contraception and Abortion from the Ancient World to the Renaissance*. Cambridge: Mass.: Harvard University Press, 1992.

Ross, Andrew. "The Ecology of Images." *The South Atlantic Quarterly* 91, no. 1 (Winter 1992).

Roszak, Theodore. *The Voice of the Earth.* New York: Simon and Schuster, 1992.

Rothman, Barbara Katz. *The Tentative Pregnancy.* New York: Viking, 1986.

Rothman, Sheila M. *Woman's Proper Place: A History of Changing Ideals and Practices, 1870 to the Present.* New York: Basic Books, 1978.

Rowland, Robyn. *Living Laboratories: Women and Reproductive Technologies.* Bloomington: Indiana University Press, 1992.

Ruddick, Sara. *Maternal Thinking: Toward a Politics of Peace.* Boston: Beacon Press, 1989.

Ruether, Rosemary Radford. *Sexism and God-Talk: Toward a Feminist Theology.* Boston: Beacon Press, 1983.

Ryan, Mary. *Motherhood in America,* 2d ed. Philadelphia: Franklin and Watts, 1978.

Sahlins, Marshall. *Stone Age Economics.* Chicago: Aldine, 1972.

Saxton, Marsha. "Born and Unborn: The Implications of Reproductive Technologies for People with Disabilities." In *Test-Tube Women: What Future for Motherhood?* edited by Rita Arditti, Renata Duelli Klein, and Shelly Minden. London: Pandora Press, 1984.

Scott, Dr. Jocelynne A. "Book Reviews." In *Reproductive and Genetic Engineering: Journal of International Feminist Analysis* 3, no. 1 (1990), p. 74.

Seegmiller, R. E., et al. "Reporting of Congenital Malformations of Utah Birth Certificates." Utah Department of Health, April 1981.

Seller, Anne. "Greenham: A Concrete Reality." *Frontiers* 8 (1985), pp. 26–31.

Sen, Gita, and Caren Grown. *Development, Crises, and Alternative Visions: Third World Women's Perspectives.* New York: Monthly Review Press, 1987.

Sen, Ilina, ed. *A Space Within the Struggle: Women's Participation in Peace Movements.* New Delhi: Kali for Women, 1990.

Shapiro, Thomas M. *Population Control Politics: Women, Sterilization, and Reproductive Choice.* Philadelphia: Temple University Press, 1985.

Sathyamala, C. Nirmala Sundharam, and Nalini Bhand. *Taking Sides: The Choices before the Health Worker.* Delhi: Bukprint, 1986.

SHIVA, VANDANA. *Staying Alive: Women, Ecology, and Development*. New Delhi: Kali for Women, 1988.

———. *The Violence of the Green Revolution: Ecological Development and Political Conflict in Punjab*. New Delhi, 1989.

SHULMAN, SETH. *The Threat at Home: Confronting the Toxic Legacy of the U.S. Military*. Boston: Beacon Press, 1992.

SIEGEL, RICHARD, MICHAEL STRASSFELD, AND SHARON STRASSFELD, EDS. *The First Jewish Catalog*. Philadelphia: The Jewish Publication Society of America, 1973.

SIMON, JULIAN L. *The Ultimate Resource*. Princeton: Princeton University Press, 1981.

SJOO, MONICA, AND BARBARA MOR. *The Great Cosmic Mother: Rediscovering the Religion of the Earth*. San Francisco: Harper and Row, 1987.

SMITH, DOROTHY E. *The Every Day World as Problematic*. Boston: Northeastern University Press, 1987.

SMITH, J. DAVID, AND K. RAY NELSON. *The Sterilization of Carrie Buck*. New Jersey: New Horizon Press, 1989.

SMITH-ROSENBERG, CAROL. *Disorderly Conduct*. New York: Oxford University Press, 1985.

SPALLONE, PATRICIA, AND DEBORAH LYNN STEINBERG, EDS. *Made to Order: The Myth of Reproductive and Genetic Progress*. New York: Pergamon Press, The Athene Series, 1987.

SPELMAN, ELIZABETH V. *Inessential Woman: Problems of Exclusion in Feminist Thought*. Boston: Beacon Press, 1988.

SPIVAK, GAYATRI CHAKRAVORTY. *In Other Words: Essays in Cultural Politics*. New York: Methuen, 1987.

SPRETNAK, CHARLENE, AND FRITJOF CAPRA. *Green Politics*. New York: Dutton, 1984.

SPRETNAK, CHARLENE. *The Politics of Women's Spirituality: Essays on the Rise of Spiritual Power within the Feminist Movement*. Garden City, N.Y.: Doubleday, 1981.

———. *The Spiritual Dimension of Green Politics*. Santa Fe: Bear, 1986.

———. *Lost Goddesses of Early Greece: A Collection of Pre-Hellenic Myths*. Boston: Beacon Press, 1981.

SRIVINAS, K. RAVI, AND A. K. KANAKAMALU. "Introducing Norplant: The Politics of Coercion." *Economic and Political Weekly* (July 18, 1992), pp. 1531–33.

STANWORTH, MICHELLE, ED. *Reproductive Technologies: Gender, Motherhood and Medicine*. Minneapolis: University of Minnesota Press, 1987.

STARHAWK. *Dreaming the Dark: Magic, Sex and Politics.* Boston: Beacon Press, 1982.

STARHAWK. "Power, Authority, and Mystery: Ecofeminism and Earth-based Spirituality." In *Reweaving the World: The Emergence of Ecofeminism,* edited by Irene Diamond and Gloria Feman Orenstein. San Francisco: Sierra Club, 1990.

STARR, PAUL. *The Social Transformation of American Medicine.* New York: Basic Books, 1982.

STEINBROOK ROBERT. "In California, Voluntary Mass Prenatal Screening." *Hastings Center Report* (October 1986), pp. 4–7.

STRASSFELD, SHARON, AND MICHAEL STRASSFELD, EDS. *The Third Jewish Catalog.* Philadelphia: The Jewish Publication Society of America, 1980.

STRATHERN, MARILYN. *Reproducing the Future: Anthropology, Kinship, and the New Reproductive Technologies.* New York: Routledge, 1992.

SUMMEY, PAMELA S., AND MARSHA HURST. "Ob/Gyn on the Rise: The Evolution of Professional Ideology in the Twentieth Century." *Women and Health* 11 (Summer 1986), pp. 103–22.

TEISH, LUISAH. *Jambalaya: The Natural Woman's Book.* San Francisco: Harper, 1985.

The New Our Bodies Ourselves. The Boston Women's Health Book Collective. New York: Simon and Schuster, 1992.

TRASK, HAUNANI-KAY. *Eros and Power: The Promise of Feminist Theory.* Philadelphia: University of Pennsylvania Press, 1986.

UNGER, ROBERTO MANGABEIRA. *Knowledge and Politics.* New York: The Free Press, 1975.

U.S. Office of Technology Assessment. *Infertility: Medical and Social Choices.* Washington D.C.: U.S. Government Printing Office, May 1988.

VAN ESTERIK, PEGGY. *Beyond the Breast-Bottle Controversy.* New Brunswick, N.J.: Rutgers University Press, 1989.

VISVANATHAN, SHIV. "Mrs. Brundtland's Disenchanted Cosmos." *Alternatives: Social Transformation and Humane Governance* 16, no. 3 (Summer 1991), pp. 377–384.

WALKER, ALICE. *In Search of Our Mother's Gardens.* San Diego: Harcourt Brace Jovanovich, 1983.

WARREN, KAREN. "Feminism and Ecology Making Connections." *Environmental Ethics* 9, no. 1 (1987).

WARWICK, DONALD. *Bitter Pills: Population Policies and their*

Implementation in Eight Developing Countries. Cambridge: Cambridge University Press, 1982.

WERTZ, RICHARD W., AND DOROTHY C. WERTZ. *Lying In: A History of Childbirth in America.* New York: Schocken, 1977.

WRESTLING, A., ED. *Environmental Warfare: A Technical, Legal and Policy Appraisal.* London: Taylor and Francis, 1984.

WESTOFF, CHARLES. "The Fertility of the American Population." In *Population: The Vital Revolution,* edited by Ronald Friedman. Garden City: Doubleday, 1964.

WHARTON, P., ET AL. "Infertility in Male Pesticide Workers." *Lancet* (1977), pp. 1259–61.

WHITMAN, WALT. *Leaves of Grass.* San Francisco: Chandler, 1968.

WHORTON, M. DONALD, ET AL. "Reproductive Hazards." In *Occupational Health: Recognizing and Preventing Work Related Disease,* edited by Barry S. Levy and David H. Wegman. Boston: Little Brown, 1983.

WICHTERICH, CHRISTA. "From the Struggle Against 'Overpopulation' to the Industrialization of Human Production." *Issues in Reproductive and Genetic Engineering* 1, no. 1 (1988), pp. 21–30.

WILLIAMS, TERRY TEMPEST. *Refuge: An Unnatural History of Family and Place.* New York: Random House, 1991.

WOLFE-DEVINE, CELIA. "Is Support for Abortion Essential to Feminism?" *New Oxford Review* (November 1990), p. 12.

World Commission on Environment and Development. *Our Common Future.* Oxford: Oxford University Press, 1987.

XENOS, NICHOLAS. *Scarcity and Modernity.* New York: Routledge, 1989.

ZOPF, PAUL E., JR. *American Women in Poverty.* New York: Greenwood Press, 1989.

INDEX